CANCER: A G...
AND THEIR FAMILIES

CANCER:

A GUIDE FOR PATIENTS AND THEIR FAMILIES

Chris and Sue Williams

A Wiley Medical Publication

JOHN WILEY & SONS

Chichester · New York · Brisbane · Toronto · Singapore

Cover illustration by Joanna Williams.

Library of Congress Cataloging-in-Publication Data:
Williams, C. J. (Christopher John Hacon)
  Cancer: A guide for patients and their families.
(A Wiley medical publication)
Includes index.
    1. Cancer—Popular works.   I. Williams, Sue.
II. Title.   III. Series.   [DNLM: 1. Medical Oncology—
popular works. QZ 201 W722c]
RC263.W494 1986   616.99'4//86–21
ISBN 0 471 91017 1 (pbk.)

British Library Cataloguing in Publication Data:
Williams, Chris, 1946–
  Cancer : A guide for patients and their families.
  1. Cancer
  I. Title   II. Williams, Sue
  616.99'4   RC261
ISBN 0 471 91017 1

Printed and Bound in Great Britain.

Contents

Preface

This book is a companion to *All about Cancer, a Practical Guide to Cancer Care*. It is shorter, and less detailed, but none the less contains the same information and advice, some of it updated. It discusses all the aspects of care, treatment, and investigations you will need to know about to understand the course of the disease. At the end of the book there is a list of societies you may wish to contact.

We hope that you will find this book interesting, informative, and a useful aid for anyone involved with cancer.

CHAPTER 1

What is cancer?

Cancer is not only a frightening disease — it is also surprisingly common. Most of us associate it with slow painful death even though many cancers can be cured and uncontrollable pain is rare. But the really frightening thing about cancer is the silence and 'taboo' that surrounds it. With this in mind the first part of the book discusses what cancer is all about and what causes it. This is followed by sections on diagnosis of cancer and the treatment of individual tumours. The last part of the book talks about the treatment of symptoms and the emotional upsets caused by the disease.

Because most of us feel that cancer means certain death we prefer to bury our heads in the sand about the subject — unless it affects us personally. Then we wonder what has gone wrong and how it started. It is difficult to give a clear answer, but this chapter aims to give a simple explanation.

Normal tissues in the body are made up of individual building blocks or cells that can divide and multiply. This ability is controlled so that cell death and cell birth are roughly equal in an adult. In a cancer the control mechanisms that maintain this balance are lost and there is uncontrolled growth of cancer cells at rates which exceed the death of normal cells in that tissue. The tumour which is formed by the cancer cells continues to grow at the expense of the patient. It may invade local tissues, or spread to nearby structures or even to distant organs. It is the invasion by local tumour or its distant spread that can cause symptoms or eventually death. Cancer is, therefore, the *uncontrolled growth of cells that will, if not stopped, spread locally or to other parts of the body*.

One of the commonest questions a patient with cancer asks is 'Why have I got cancer; why me?' When cancer is diagnosed many patients are more concerned with *why* the tumour has occurred than what can be done about it.

1

There are probably many causes, and more than one may be needed to produce each individual tumour. Most cancers are caused by exposure to chemicals (called carcinogens: substances that can cause cancer), though such carcinogens are not necessarily man-made, but may be around us in our natural environment (Table 1). They affect cells by altering the normal DNA (DNA is the genetic material that controls cell function) in the centre or nucleus of the cell. The damage can be repaired, may cause the cell to die or may produce no detectable change. Occasionally, however, it may cause cancer.

Carcinogens act silently and frequently do not produce cancer for many years (an interval known as the latent period which may be as long as twenty or more years).

Viruses have been shown to cause cancer in some animals but so far they have not been proved to do so in humans. Despite this it is likely that some cancers in man are due to viruses. However, they do not cause epidemics of cancer as a complicated set of circumstances is needed before a cancer is produced by the virus. AIDS is a very special situation in which a virus damages the immune system; this in turn may result in

Table 1 Estimated causes of human cancers	
Cause	Estimated proportion of cancer deaths in Western countries* (%)
Environmental	
Cigarette smoking	35
Diet	30
Occupation	2
Background radiation	2
Non-environmental	
Genetic	5
Total	74
Unaccounted for	26

*This estimate is based on figures from the United States.

development of cancers of the immune system itself, as well as unusual infections.

There are other causes of cancer, some known (like radiation) and others unknown. Table 1 lists these and estimates how much influence each factor exerts. It is obvious that the only one easily changed is smoking.

CHAPTER 2

Who gets cancer?

People most likely to develop cancer fall into one of several groups at risk.

INHERITED CANCERS

There is no inherited risk of cancer for most people. However, in some families it does seem to be passed on from generation to generation.

Cancer families

There are some families with a very high incidence of certain cancers. The commonest tumours in these families are those of the large bowel, womb (uterus), stomach and breast. They tend to occur at an unusually early age and may develop in several places at once. These patients have a *very* strong family history (over several generations) of cancers and if this is part of your family pattern it is wise to be alert for symptoms and contact your family doctor if you are at all suspicious.

Polyposis coli and Gardener's syndrome

These are inherited conditions in which there are many (often hundreds) of polyps in the large bowel. These polyps (fleshy outgrowths) are harmless but may become cancerous. Multiple polyps usually develop by the age of 20 and can be detected by a special X-ray, a barium enema (page 31). As the risk of cancer is so very high it is usually advised that an operation is done to remove the large bowel before a tumour can develop. This means having a ileostomy (bringing the bowel to the surface of the abdomen) (page 290), something very difficult for a young person to adjust to. However, the alternative is an almost certain chance of bowel cancer by the age of 40. Remember that a ileostomy is *not* required for the vast number of people who have a few polyps in the large bowel. After taking them out (using a sigmoidoscope or colonoscope) (page 59) patients will just be monitored with intermittent tests.

Ulcerative colitis

Those who have chronic ulcerative colitis, which is not an inherited condition, have an increased risk of cancer of the large bowel which becomes very pronounced after the ulcerative colitis has been active for 10 or more years. For those with longstanding colitis it is usual to remove the large bowel in order to avoid the increasing risk of cancer. A ileostomy (page 290) is usually performed (bowel brought up to the abdominal wall) though in some cases surgeons argue that the small bowel can be connected to the rectum. The rectum is then examined *regularly* (by a sigmoidoscope — page 59) so that any sign of cancer can be detected early. This approach is, however, not accepted by many doctors,as it still allows a small risk of cancer.

Stomach cancer

People with the blood disorder pernicious anaemia have an increased risk of developing stomach cancer. Some doctors suggest routine check-ups though this is not of any proven benefit.

Breast cancer

In Western societies breast cancer is very common and it may run in families. Those women whose immediate female relatives have early breast cancer (before 40 years) or cancer of both breasts, have a higher than usual risk of developing breast cancer themselves. Although routine self-examination of the breast is recommended for all women (Chapter 5), those at high risk because of their family history should be seen by their doctor for a routine check-up from their early twenties. After the age of 30, routine mammograms are *probably* advisable.

Skin cancer

The commonest reason for most types of skin cancer is excessive exposure to sunlight. However, there are several rare inherited causes of skin cancers. (1) Xeroderma pigmentosa is an inherited condition in which the skin is unable to repair the damage caused by sunlight and multiple cancers develop. Protective measures to reduce exposure to sunlight will reduce the risk of cancers. (2) Albinism. This is the inherited condition in which there is a lack of pigment in the skin, hair, and iris of the eye. Such people are very sensitive to sunlight and have a high incidence of skin cancer; avoidance of sunlight reduces the risk. (3) Neurofibromatosis. This is a rare inherited condition in which there are soft fleshy skin tags, brownish patches all over the skin and outgrowths on some nerves. These areas may undergo a cancerous change in about one in every 14 people with the condition. (4) Malignant melanoma (malignant mole). This is a tumour of the pigment cells in the skin. It starts when a mole changes its character, it either grows, darkens, or bleeds and it does occasionally run in families, so that there may be an inherited predisposition to the tumour. It is more common in white people who get sunburnt.

Eye tumours

Retinoblastoma. This is a rare cancer of the back of the eye (retina). It develops early in life and in about half the cases is inherited. This type often occurs in both eyes and in families with such a history, children should have a regular eye examination in childhood.

Other inherited tumours

Although there are a number of other tumours that run in families they are all fortunately rare.

OCCUPATIONAL RISK OF CANCER

Some jobs carry a risk of cancer because they expose workers to chemicals that can cause cancer. Employees often find it difficult to get information about the risks associated with their job, this is often due to an inability to accurately define which jobs carry a risk of cancer as well as to a reluctance on the part of employers to openly discuss the potential risks that they are exposed to. If you are worried about risks at work it is worth asking your company doctor about it.

ENVIRONMENTAL CAUSES OF CANCER

Everyone may be exposed to carcinogens in their everyday life. Although there has been a lot of worry about food additives and other chemicals, none has been *definitely* shown to cause cancer.

LIFE STYLE

Some cancers may be related to the way we live and consequent exposure to carcinogens.

Lung cancer

It is not necessary to say too much about the effects of cigarette smoking beyond confirming that it is the most important carcinogen that we know of and that many thousands of cases of lung cancer a year could be avoided; this is in addition to the even greater risks of heart and blood vessel diseases.

Cervical cancer

This risk of developing cancer of the cervix (neck of the womb) appears to be related to sexual intercourse. Cervical cancer is most common in women who start having intercourse at an early age and with many different partners. Cervical cancer *may* be caused by a virus infecting the vagina and cervix. The introduction of cervical smears has meant that many more of these cancers are picked up at an early stage or when the condition is pre-malignant (page 12). Routine pelvic examinations and a cervical smear ought to be done in women when they become sexually active.

Skin cancer

Most skin cancers are related to exposure to sunlight. Sun tan may be attractive but unfortunately there is an increased risk of various types of skin cancer if exposure is excessive.

Obesity

Overweight women have a higher risk of developing both breast and uterine (womb) cancer which may be due to hormonal changes caused by obesity.

Testicular cancer

The only known predisposing cause of testicular cancer is failure of the testis to descend into the scrotum. The testes develop in the abdomen and move downwards, reaching the scrotum just before birth and if this fails to happen (an undescended testicle) the risk of subsequent cancer of the testis is increased fifty-fold. It has become usual to operate and bring the testis into the scrotum before the age of 5 years if it has not descended. This was thought to prevent cancer from developing but it seems likely that the damage is done and cancer may still develop. Some surgeons now remove the abnormal testis (which usually does not work, anyway) to stop any risk of cancer. Men with one testis are sexually normal and can father children.

Although most patients with an undescended testicle do not develop cancer, surgery to bring the testis into the scrotum is the least that should be done, as a tumour developing within the abdomen will not cause symptoms till an advanced stage.

CHAPTER 3

Which are the common cancers?

It depends on which part of the world you live in as to which cancers are most common, but the commonest cancers in Britain

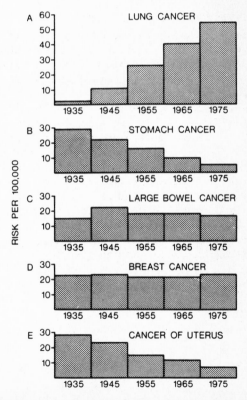

Figure 1 Changes in the frequency of common tumours during the years 1935–1975. Some became more common (especially lung), others were seen less often (stomach and uterus) whilst the risk of breast and bowel cancer changed little

Table 2 Number of new cases of cancer per 100,000 people

Type (site) of tumour in order of frequency	Number of cancers/100,000 per year	
	Male	Female
Lung	70	13
Uterus (womb)	—	76
Breast	1	75
Colon	34	30
Prostate	59	—
Rectum	17	11
Bladder	22	6
Lymphomas	16	10
Stomach	16	7
Pancreas	12	7
Leukaemias	12	7
Mouth	11	4
Ovary	—	14
Nervous system	7	5
Kidney	8	4
Larynx (voice box)	9	1
Oesophagus (gullet)	6	2

are those of the lung, breast, large bowel, prostate, uterus and stomach. A more complete list is shown in Table 2.

The overall incidence of cancer, taking into account that people are living longer, has not really increased in the past fifty years; although some tumours have become more common, others have become less common (Figure 1).

CHAPTER 4

What are the warning signs of cancer?

An early diagnosis of cancer is very important. Most cancers grow from a single cell and eventually spread to other parts of the body. The smaller a tumour when it is discovered, the greater is the chance that it has not spread.

It is vital to notice warning signs of cancer in order to pick up a tumour early. The following symptoms are a reason for consulting a doctor immediately. None of them automatically means cancer but a careful examination is needed to rule it out.

Many people dislike consulting their own doctor with seemingly trivial symptoms but they should be taken seriously and no doctor will ever think that his time is being wasted. So make an appointment immediately if you have any of the following:

Breast   Lump or thickening in breast, discharge from the nipple.

Colon and rectum   Change in bowel habit, rectal bleeding.

Lung   Persistent cough, lingering chest infection, or coughing up blood.

Mouth, throat and larynx (voice box)   Sore that does not heal, difficulty in swallowing or change in voice.

Skin   Sore that does not heal or change in wart or mole, bleeding from mole.

Uterus (womb) **and cervix**   Any bleeding between normal periods or, after menopause, any bleeding at all, or any unusual discharge.

Kidney or bladder   Pain or difficulty passing urine or blood in the urine.

Stomach   Indigestion, difficulty in swalliing or persistent vomiting.

CHAPTER 5

Cancer screening

If the treatment of cancer is most successful when a tumour is very small then it makes sense to use special tests to detect tumours before they cause any symptoms. Cancer screening is a relatively recent idea and the assumption that it will improve the care of cancer remains unproven for many tumours.

Screening tests have been mainly concerned with a few common tumours and we will concentrate on these. Doctors do not all agree on the need for screening and trials testing the usefulness and assessing the cost and benefits of various types of screening are being carried out.

Cancer of the cervix (neck of the womb)

In many Western countries deaths from cervical cancer have reduced by up to 50 per cent in the past 20 years. During this time there has been increasing awareness of the importance of early diagnosis and a concentrated effort to screen for the disease using the cervical smear (page 59).

Cells from the cervix are examined under a microscope after they have been scraped from the lining of the cervix. Many of the cancers found by this method are localized to the surface and are called *in situ* cancers. Cervical cancer, when caught at this stage, is nearly always curable (more than 95 per cent). It is important to have routine smear tests done as tests performed when a woman has symptoms of cervical cancer are much more likely to show an invasive tumour which is more difficult to cure. In some women *pre*-malignant cells (cells that may turn into cancer cells) are seen and these women should have regular screening to check if the smear is becoming more abnormal.

There are no universally accepted guide-lines on when the tests should be started and how often they should be done. Ideally tests should probably be started at 25 years of age and be repeated annually, though some doctors will allow gaps of up to 3 years after two negative tests. Patients with abnormal vaginal bleeding or a persistent vaginal discharge should probably have a smear every 6 months for 2 years. Women with abnormal pre-malignant cells (called dysplastic) will need to have a biopsy of the cervix and, if available, direct microscopic examination (colposcopy). If there is no sign of cancer they should be followed with further cervical smears at 6-monthly intervals.

While the results of treatment of *in situ* cancers detected by smear are very good it has less impact if it picks up more advanced cancer. The problem of this cancer is far from settled and even the role of mass screening is still being investigated. However, doctors agree that all women should have routine smears. The main problem with screening is that those women at greatest risk often do not come for the test.

Breast cancer

Breast cancer is the commonest cancer in British women. The breast is easily examined and there has been great interest in persuading women to undertake routine examination for breast lumps. Screening examination can be of three types:

(1) The simplest is self-examination of the breast (Figure 2). This is the first line of screening and a careful examination should pick up small lumps. Women still having their periods need to examine their breasts at the same time each month as the shape and feel of the breasts changes with the menstrual cycle. The best time to examine the breasts is 7 days after the start of each period.
(2) Breast examination by a doctor or specially trained nurse. This may be done annually.
(3) Mammography. This is a special X-ray of the breast, useful for detecting cancers too small to be felt.

The latter two methods are often only available in special screening clinics. Various 'Well Women' clinics have been set up around Britain which carry out routine regular screening programmes. Check if there is one in your area.

All patients with a breast lump should be seen by a specialist

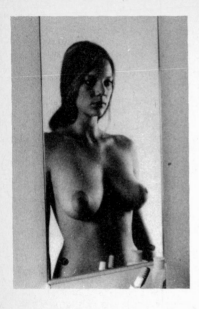

1. Undress to the waist and sit or stand in front of a mirror in a good light with your arms comfortably by your sides. If sitting, you may find it preferable to rest your hands lightly on your hips. Look at your breasts carefully. In the first examination you should note the normal size and shape of each breast and the position of the nipples so that you will be aware of any changes that might develop. In subsequent examinations you should look for any inequality in the size or shape of your breasts. Pay special attention to any alterations in the surface of the breast, such as a swelling, skin puckering (dimple), rash, discolouration or very prominent veins. Note whether either nipple is retracted (turned in).

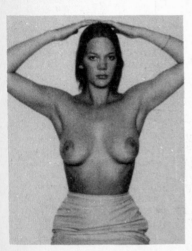

2. Now place the hands lightly on the top of the head and again look at the breasts carefully, concentrating especially on the nipples. This position will emphasize any difference in size or shape between the two breasts. Look particularly for any excessive upward or outward movement of either nipple.

Figure 2 Breast self-examination (reproduced, with permission, from a leaflet produced by The Women's National Cancer Control Campaign of 1 South Audley Street, London W1. International copyright of the Women's National Cancer Control Campaign)

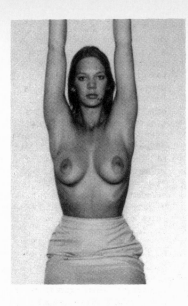

3. Momentarily stretch the arms above the head. Again this will emphasize any difference between the two breasts.

4. Now place the hands firmly on your hips and when you are comfortable, push inwards towards the hips. You should feel the muscles on the upper part of your chest beneath your breasts tighten when you do this. Look at the breasts carefully while you keep pressing. This movement will emphasize any puckering of the skin or any abnormal retraction of either nipple. Remember to look at the under surface of the breast during this part of the examination. It is often easier to stand up to do this properly. You have completed the INSPECTION part of the examination and it is now time to feel for any abnormal lumps in the breasts. Again it is important at the first examination to note the normal consistency of your breasts, so that you will be aware of any change in subsequent examinations. Many women who have not yet reached the change of life normally have rather lumpy breasts just before the period and in some this may persist throughout the whole month. This may cause uncertainty at first, but with each successive examination it should become easier to decide whether any unusual lump is present.

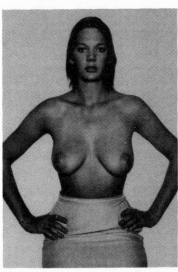

16

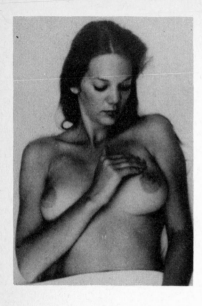

5. Lie down comfortably on a firm surface with your head on a pillow. Place a folded towel under the shoulder slightly raising the side that you are going to examine first. The left breast is felt with your right hand and vice versa. The first part of the examination is done with the arm by the side. Feel with the flat of the pads of the middle three fingers. The fingers should be kept straight but the hand flexible. Each time you feel, the breast tissue should be pressed towards the chest wall. Firm but gentle pressure should be used.

6.7.8. The examination starts just above the nipple and continues outward in a spiral fashion around the breast. EVERY PART of the breast must be felt so that two or three complete circles will need to be made depending on the size of the breast. Any unusual discrete lump or nodule should be noted.

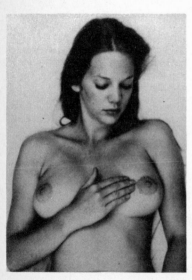

Figure 2 (*contd*). Breast self-examination

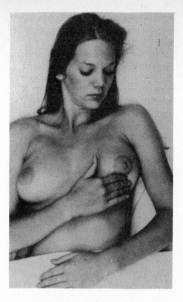

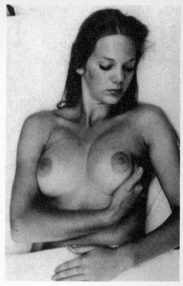

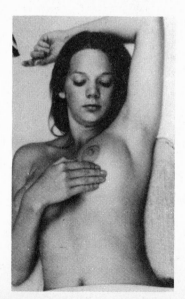

9. It is not easy to examine the outermost part of the breast with the arm by the side. When you have completed the first series of circular movements place the arm comfortably above the head with the elbow bent. Repeat the examination of all the breast now, paying especial attention to the outer part which can now be felt with more certainty. Never rush palpation of the breasts which must be done slowly, gently, and thoroughly.

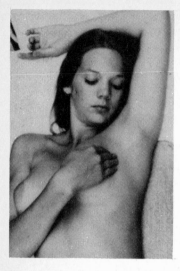

10. The final part of the examination is of the so-called tail of the breast which extends towards the armpit. This can only be examined properly with the arm above the head.

You have now completed palpation of one breast and this must be repeated for the other side.

Having completed self-examination of your breasts you will have decided whether they remain unchanged or whether any unusual feature has appeared. To remind you of these features, they are again listed below.

Warning Signs

ON INSPECTION

Unusual difference in size or shape of the breasts.

Alterations in the position of either nipple.

Retraction (turning in) of either nipple.

Puckering (dimple) of the skin surface.

Unusual rash on the breast or nipple.

Unusual prominence of the veins over either breast.

ON PALPATION

Unusual discrete lump or nodule in any part of either breast.

Routine Examinations

Try to make the examination of your breasts a monthly habit. Immediately following a period would be a suitable time, or on the first day of the month if you have had the menopause.

Figure 2 (*contd*). Breast self-examination

so that it may be carefully examined and if necessary biopsied. The majority of breast lumps that are biopsied do not contain cancer (they are benign), but this cannot be shown without looking at the lump under a microscope. The decision, whether to perform a biopsy or not, can only be made by a specialist and general practitioners should refer all patients with a breast lump immediately to a breast clinic.

Cancer of the large bowel (colon and rectum)

The benefits of screening for cancer of the large bowel are less clear. It is common in Britain and the outlook after surgical removal of the cancer is related to the extent of spread. Early diagnosis might improve survival in this tumour. Most patients present with symptoms of constipation, diarrhoea, or rectal bleeding, though harmless polyps may also cause similar symptoms.

Nearly all cancers of the bowel bleed (90 per cent) and testing of the stools for blood (occult blood testing) has been used to screen for cancer. The place of occult blood tests and examination of the bowel using a sigmoidoscope or colonoscopy for screening is not clear, though it is not usually recommended in this country.

Prostate cancer

Prostate cancer becomes more common after the age of 50 years. The prostate can be felt during a rectal examination and any abnormal lump or nodule detected. If a routine annual physical examination is done this should include a rectal examination.

Cancers of the mouth

Cancers of the mouth and throat can often be seen or felt. A routine dental visit (at least annually) should allow early detection of many of these tumours. Dentists, in addition to looking after a patient's teeth, will always examine the soft parts of your mouth.

Cancer of the uterus (womb)

Cancer of the uterus is not reliably diagnosed by a cervical smear. The only sure way to detect uterine cancer is by a D and C (D and C stands for dilation and curettage, this is the scraping away of the lining of the uterus, under general anaesthetic, for microscopic examination). If a D and C is done you will need to be admitted to hospital for a short period.

These tests are, therefore, not used to screen for cancer. Any abnormal vaginal bleeding is an indication for investigation and frequently a D and C is done to be sure that there is no uterine cancer.

Lung cancer

Screening chest X-rays have not been shown to improve the survival changes of most people with lung cancer. This is because lung cancer has usually spread before it can be seen on a routine chest X-ray.

Malignant melanoma

In Australia, where malignant melanoma is a very common skin cancer, special clinics for early diagnosis have been set up. Patients with skin lumps or moles that are changing are encouraged to come to these clinics and tumours are being recognized at an earlier stage — when the chance for cure is greatest.

CHAPTER 6

How is the diagnosis made?

Although a doctor may suspect cancer, a diagnosis cannot be made without examining a piece of the suspicious tissue under a microscope. A biopsy (removal of a piece of tissue for examination — by a small operation or by a needle) **must** be done if cancer is suspected. For details on how biopsies are performed see Chapter 10 and the chapters on each of the common tumours.

When a biopsy has been taken the tissue is prepared and stained with special dyes for examination under a microscope.

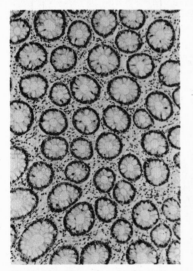

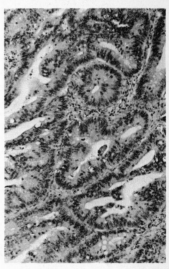

Figure 3(a) Normal stomach tissue: this microscopic view shows a regular appearance of symmetrical glands

Figure 3(b) Cancer of the stomach: this microscopic view (taken from the same patient as Figure 3(a)) shows that the glandular structure is grossly changed and that the cells making up the glands are different

The doctor (a pathologist) looking at the biopsy can tell if a cancer is present by the disruption of the normal pattern of the tissue and its cells (Figure 3). The pathologist will usually be certain if there is cancer and may be able to say where it has come from or if it has spread from somewhere else. Some types of cancer, however, may be difficult to detect and special tests may be needed, or even another biopsy, to be sure of the diagnosis.

CHAPTER 7

How does cancer spread?

One of the biggest problems with cancer is that it may spread to other areas of the body. Despite advances in surgical technique and anaesthetics, apparent complete surgical removal of a tumour is, in fact, often incomplete. Tumours frequently recur at the site they were taken away from, in nearby structures, or at other parts of the body.

Failure of surgery or radiotherapy to cure tumours is often due to spread of the cancer before treatment is even started, and an understanding of the ways that cancer may spread is clearly essential to planning treatment. Unfortunately our knowledge is limited; apart from a simple understanding of the routes of spread we do not know why or how each type of cancer spreads in the way it does.

ROUTES OF SPREAD

Local invasion

Most tumours continue to grow at the site where they originally developed. Some will invade nearby parts of the body and this may include spread of the cancer into major organs such as the bladder or bowel in the abdomen or into bones. Such invasion may cause pain, especially if the growth is into bone or local nerves and many of the early symptoms of cancer may be caused by this type of spread.

Lymphatic spread

The lymph system is a fine network of vessels, like blood vessels, whose job is to remove excess fluid and unwanted substances such as bacteria from the body's tissues. If a tumour invades locally into these abundant lymph vessels it may spread along them to nearby lymph nodes. Lymph nodes, (or glands) are pea-sized nodules scattered in various parts of the body.

Their function is to filter out foreign material and to produce lymphocytes (a type of immune cell in the blood). As a result the lymph node traps the cancer cells in the lymph fluid and cancer grows within the node.

As the pattern of lymphatic drainage from most parts of the body is known, doctors' examine the draining lymph nodes for enlargement and the initial treatment plan may include therapy to these lymph nodes. Progressive spread along lymph vessels and nodes may occur so that quite distant lymph glands may become involved.

Distant spread by the bloodstream

If tumour invades a blood vessel then cancer cells may break off into the bloodstream and be carried to other parts of the body. As blood vessels become progressively smaller these cells become trapped and the cancer may then develop at that point. The pattern of spread depends on the direction of the blood flow from the original tumour. The veins draining the bowel pass the blood on to the liver. Veins from the rest of the body drain into the lungs. Thus the major site of spread in cases of bowel cancer is the liver. The lungs are the commonest site of metastases in other tumours though secondary liver involvement and spread to many other organs in the body are also common. The pattern of spread of individual tumours is discussed in the chapters on the major types of tumours.

Avoiding recurrence of a tumour

(a) It is essential that there is a rim or margin of normal tissue surrounding a tumour when it is removed. If tumour is present in the margin around the lump removed then the cancer is likely to recur at that site. All surgical specimens should be examined to be sure that there is a tumour-free margin.

(b) Lymph nodes draining the tumour should be examined during an operation and by special X-rays. If there is evidence of spread to adjacent lymph nodes treatment for all the draining lymph nodes should be included in the initial treatment plan.

(c) Some tumours commonly spread by the blood to other

parts of the body. Tests to see if spread has occurred (see next chapter) should normally be done before therapy is started as the presence of secondary tumour (metastases) may alter the treatment plan.

CHAPTER 8

What is staging?

When the diagnosis of cancer has been made it is important to know whether the cancer has spread (see chapter 7) before treatment is planned. This is called 'staging' as the degree of spread of a tumour is often referred to, by doctors, at the 'stage' which it has reached.

The importance of staging lies in the different types of treatment that are available. Both surgery and radiotherapy are 'local' treatments. They are only effective when the tumour has not spread beyond the area where it arose or its draining lymph nodes (see page 22). Drug therapy (chemotherapy) is the mainstay of treatment when the tumour is widespread. Accurate staging is important in choosing the most effective treatment and also for avoiding unnecessary therapy. Patients found to have metastatic disease (distant spread) can be saved from extensive surgery or radiotherapy that would not be useful.

The main aims of staging are to estimate:

(a) How large is the original tumour? Does it invade into surrounding normal tissues?

(b) Has the tumour spread to nearby draining lymph nodes?

(c) Is there evidence of spread of cancer to other parts of the body (metastases)?

The tests used to stage different tumours vary enormously. A brief discussion of the type of tests carried out for the common cancers are included in the chapters on individual tumours and details of the way the major tests are carried out are given in the next chapter.

For many tumour types there are special **staging classifications** that are used to describe the extent of spread of that particular tumour. These are discussed in some of the sections on the individual tumours.

CHAPTER 9

Investigations used to diagnose and stage cancer

The major problem that doctors face when examining a patient is an inability to see what is actually going on inside the body. By taking an accurate detailed history, feeling (palpation), listening with a stethoscope, and testing the body's functions (i.e. testing reflexes) a physician gains information that helps make a diagnosis. Over the last fifty years a new branch of medicine has grown up that uses special techniques to examine the inside

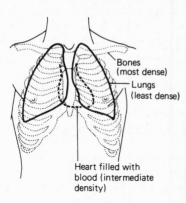

Figure 4(a) Diagrammatic representation of the structures of the chest as they show up on an X-ray. Bone is most dense, then the heart, and the lungs are least dense

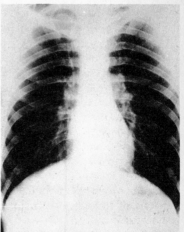

Figure 4(b) Normal chest X-ray showing how the bones, heart, and lungs are seen according to their density. The heart is dense (white) and shows up most clearly because it is so much bigger than the bones even though they are more dense. The lungs are hardly seen (very dark) as they are filled with air

of the body. Tests that will outline and show the extent of spread of a tumour are clearly of major importance and all patients with cancer will have some of the tests discussed in this section. The type and number of investigations will depend upon where the tumour started to grow. This chapter outlines some of the commoner investigations. It is important that you ask your doctor about individual tests before they are done as there may be variations in technique from hospital to hospital. Tests not included here will need to be discussed and a list of suggested questions is included at the end of the chapter.

RADIOLOGY

This is the use of X-rays to produce a photographic film which outlines the body's tissues by their density. Dense tissues (e.g. bone) absorb more X-rays than less dense structures, such as lung, and an outline of the organs by their density (Figure 4) is produced on an X-ray plate (a photographic negative). This is the basis of conventional X-rays, such as a routine chest X-ray, that we are familiar with.

Radiological tests can be divided into two broad categories.
(1) Plain films.
(2) Contrast studies.

Plain films are ordinary X-rays taken of any part of the body without special preparation or procedures. Examples are the routine chest X-ray or bone X-ray that we are all familiar with. Plain films or X-rays are of less use in examining many other parts of the body because their consistency is similar, and special ways to increase the density of the organ being examined are needed. Dyes or *contrast media* which are dense and show up clearly on X-rays are given so that the density of the structure is increased compared with the neighbouring tissues (Figure 5).

The rest of this section outlines the various types of radiological tests, with details of how they are performed, whether preparation is required, and possible side-effects.

Plain X-rays

These X-rays require no special preparation, are painless, and have no significant side-effects. In addition most X-ray depart-

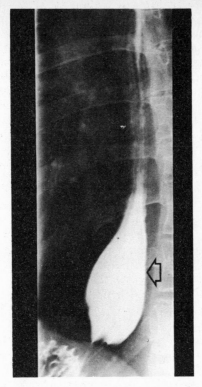

Figure 5 Barium dye outlining (see arrow) the oesophagus (gullet) in the chest

ments do not need to book plain X-rays ahead of time and are able to perform the test immediately. The time required for such X-rays is minimal.

Mammograms

- Mammograms are special plain X-rays of the breast. No special preparation is needed but talcum powder, deodorant, perfumes, or creams should not be used on the breasts during the 24 hours before the tests as they cause shadows on the X-ray film.

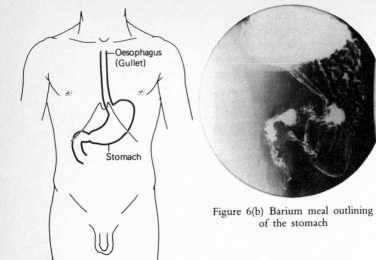

Figure 6(b) Barium meal outlining of the stomach

Figure 6(a) Diagramamtic representation of the upper part of the gastrointestinal tract

- Women strip to the waist and the breast to be X-rayed is placed on a small platform and a cone shaped device gently compresses the breast. An X-ray of both breasts is usually taken. The test takes less than one hour and afterwards patients can carry on all normal activities.

Contrast X-rays

Barium meal or swallow (upper G.I. series)

This is an investigation using *contrast material* (a barium compound) to outline the gullet (oesophagus), stomach, and upper part of the intestines.

- Patients are usually asked not to eat or drink for about 6 hours before the test: patients taking regular drugs by mouth should check with their doctor.

- The test consists of drinking up to a glassful of a white cream (the barium mixture). Some people find the taste of this unpleasant. As the barium is swallowed, the radiologist (specialist in X-ray diagnosis), is able to follow its passage into the stomach and the upper digestive system on an X-ray screen (in a darkened room). X-ray pictures will be tkaen during the examination (Figure 6); the series of films required usually means that the patient is tipped, on a mobile couch, into various positions so that the best views may be obtained. These include lying back on the couch whilst it is in the vertical position as well as lying sideways.

- If the gullet (oesophagus) alone is to be examined (barium swallow) the test should take less than half an hour. If a full barium meal examination is done, then the test is usually completed within 1½ hours. However, follow-up films the same day or occasionally on the following day may be needed in some cases. A barium meal and follow-through (an examination of the stomach and small intestine) normally requires further X-ray films for up to 6 or more hours.

- Following a barium meal patients may become constipated and pass pale stools. Constipation is more common in people who are also using medicines for pain. A laxative may be given after the test.

- Many patients are able to drive home after a barium meal, but some feel weak after the examination, particularly if they are unwell before the test, and they will need help travelling home. The major discomforts of the test are drinking the barium, which patients often dislike, and tipping the couch to obtain the best views.

Barium enema

A barium enema is a special X-ray of the lower or large bowel (*colon* and *rectum*). To prepare for this, the bowel must be absolutely clean.

- Preparation for this X-ray will vary from hospital to hospital,

Table 3 Minimal residual diet		
Type of food	Foods included	Foods excluded
Drinks	Black coffee, tea, fizzy drinks	Milk, milk drinks
Bread	Dry biscuits	All breads
Desserts	Sorbets, clear gelatin, jelly	Custards, puddings, desserts made with milk, ice-cream
Fats	Bacon, butter	Cream
Meat, poultry, fish, cheese, and eggs	Lamb, veal, chicken, turkey, whitefish, eggs	Fried meat, poultry, or fish. All cheese
Potato, pasta	Macaroni, noodles, rice, spaghetti	Potatoes
Soups	Clear soups or broths	Cream soups
Vegetables	Tomato juice only	All vegetables
Condiments and spices	Salt, small amounts of pepper	All other spices, pickles, nuts, and olives

but basically consists of:

(1) Eating a light diet for 2 days before the examination, e.g. meals of eggs, but *not* meat, fish, fruit or vegetables in any form. Patients should have plenty to drink. Table 3 shows the foods that may be eaten with a light or 'minimal residue' diet.

(2) A laxative is usually given the day before the test.

(3) Extra liquids should be drunk the day before the test and no solid food taken from the evening before the X-ray. A

Table 4 Clear liquid diet	
Type of food	Foods included
Drinks	Coffee, tea, fizzy drinks
Desserts	Sorbets, gelatin, jelly
Fruits	Fruit juices only
Soups	Clear soups, consommé, clear broth
Condiments	Salt

typical clear liquid diet is shown in Table 4. No food or drink should be taken on the morning of the investigation.

- Diabetics should not follow these instructions but should contact the doctor who is to perform the test and explain that they are diabetic. Alternative methods of preparation will be arranged.

- Before the barium enema can be done it is usual to wash to bowel out (an enema) to make sure that it is as clean as possible. After a variable period a barium mixture is run into the bowel by a tube passed into the rectum. The barium shows up on an X-ray screen (the room is darkened so the radiologist can see the screen clearly) and an outline of the large bowel is recorded on an X-ray plate (Figure 7). These days it is usual to pass some air into the lower bowel to distend it. The results of X-rays of the bowel by this method (called a double contrast barium enema) are usually much better than the old barium enema, without the air, and can pick up small abnormalities — cancerous or otherwise. When the barium and air have filled the bowel it will cause a sensation of pressure but it is important to hold the barium in the bowel till the X-rays have been finished.

- During the X-ray you may be turned or tipped (on a couch) to various positions in order to get the best view of different parts of the large bowel.

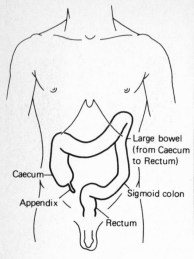

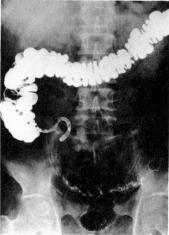

Figure 7(b) Barium enema outlining the large bowel

Figure 7(a) Diagrammatic representation of the lower part of the gastroinstinal tract

- The test takes up to 2½ hours including time for the wash-out of the bowel.
- The main problems with the test are the unpleasantness of the bowel wash-out and infusion of the barium and air.
- You may not feel like driving after the test as it may be tiring.
- Patients will, of course, pass pale stools with barium in them for some days after the test. A laxative may be prescribed in order to remove the barium as quickly as possible.

Intravenous pyelogram (IVP)

An IVP is a contrast X-ray to outline the *kidneys, the ureters* (tubes connecting the kidneys to the bladder), and the *bladder* itself.

- To obtain the best view of the kidneys it is important that

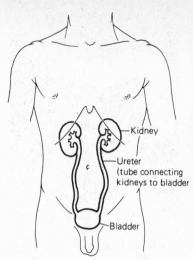

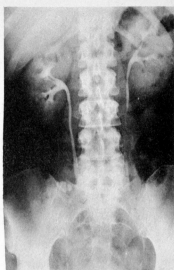

Figure 8(a) Diagrammatic representation of the kidneys, ureters, and bladder

Figure 8(b) Intravenous pyelogram showing dye outlining these structures

the overlying bowel should be cleaned out. Most hospitals therefore ask patients to take laxatives for 2 days before the test and to have a light meal the day before the test. On the day of the test you will be asked **not** to eat **or** drink. If you are diabetic you should tell the doctor arranging the test so that an appropriate diet can be arranged. Patients taking regular medicines by mouth should also check with their doctor.

- The technique of the test is to inject an X-ray contrast liquid into a vein in the forearm. This material will first appear in the kidneys and then outline the ureters and bladder (Figure 8). During the injection many patients feel hot and flushed and may be uncomfortable but this rapidly settles.

- Rarely patients may react against the dye (a type of allergic reaction). Patients becoming short of breath or feeling faint should tell the doctor giving the injection. If it is caused by a reaction this can be reversed rapidly by the use of simple drugs.

- Following the injection of the dye a series of X-rays of the abdomen are taken starting within 5 minutes and continuing for up to 1 hour.

- Occasionally a tight binder (about 25 cm wide) is placed across the abdomen to improve the X-ray view.

- It is sometimes necessary to take late X-ray pictures if the doctor wishes to follow the progress of dye which is slow to pass through a kidney.

- Occasionally it may be necessary to perform tomogram X-rays (page 44) of a kidney to get the best view.

- The test usually lasts less than 1 hour and many patients are able to drive home afterwards though some may not feel happy about this if the injection caused much flushing or discomfort.

Oral cholecystogram (gall-bladder series)

An oral cholecystogram is an X-ray taken to outline the *gall-bladder* a contrast dye having been taken by mouth.

- As with most X-rays of abdominal organs it is necessary to clean out the bowel to get the best views. Laxatives are usually given for the two nights before the test. Following a light meal, plain X-rays of the abdomen are taken and if these are satisfactory (the bowel is sufficiently clear) you will be given X-ray dye tablets to be taken at a specified time before the second part of the test.

- You should have a light breakfast (these foods are permitted: fresh vegetables — cooked without fat — fruit, lean meat, dry toast or bread, tea or coffee). The following foods must be avoided: milk, butter, cream, eggs, salad dressings, or any dairy product or foods containing fats. The tablets should be taken with water as specified and *nothing* further eaten, though water may be drunk.

- The dye in the capsules is absorbed from the stomach and is

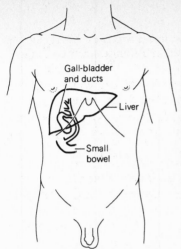

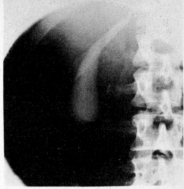

Figure 9(b) Cholecystogram showing dye outlining the gall-bladder

Figure 9(a) Diagrammatic representation of the relationship
between the liver, gall-bladder, and
small bowel

then concentrated by the liver and passes into the gall-bladder
which acts as a reservoir for the bile (Figure 9).

- The dye in the gall-bladder shows up on an X-ray of the
  abdomen. X-rays at varying times and in differing positions
  are taken to get the best view of the gall-bladder.

- It is sometimes necessary for patients to drink a little milk.
  This causes the gall-bladder to contract and squeezes the dye
  and bile into the tube (bile duct) connecting the gall-bladder
  to the bowel. It is to prevent this contraction that fatty foods
  must be avoided before the test.

- The test is frequently completed within $1\frac{1}{2}$ hours though late
  films may be required in some patients.

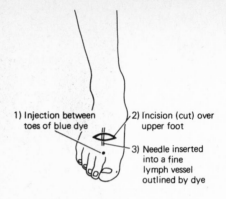

1) Injection between toes of blue dye

2) Incision (cut) over upper foot

3) Needle inserted into a fine lymph vessel outlined by dye

Figure 10 The technique used for a lymphangiogram: (1) An injection of blue dye is given between the toes. (2) When the dye has been taken up by the fine lymphatics a small incision (cut) is made over the top of the foot. (3) A fine needle is then inserted into a tiny lymph vessel and dye injected

- Most patients should be able to drive after the test as there is little discomfort and few after-effects.

Lymphangiogram

A lymphangiogram is an X-ray examination of the *lymph vessels* and *lymph nodes* of the legs and abdomen. The lymph system is a fine network of vessels, like blood vessels, which connect the lymph nodes or glands. Their function is to remove fluid or unwanted substances in the body's tissues. The test is in two parts spread over two days.

- *Day 1.* First of all your feet will be cleaned with an antiseptic. Next (Figure 10) an injection (with a small needle) of greeny-blue dye is given between the first and second toes of each foot. This dye is taken up by the fine lymph vessels over the top of each foot. Local anaesthetic is then injected to 'freeze' the skin and when this has taken effect the foot is cleaned again with alcohol and a small cut is made over the top of the foot and the small lymph vessels (now outlined by the green-blue dye) are identified. A very fine needle is passed

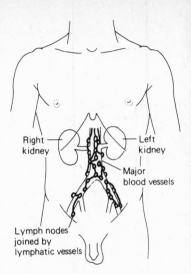

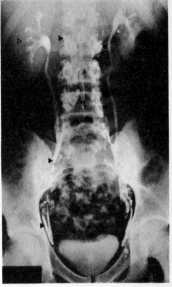

Figure 11(a) Diagrammatic representation of the lymph nodes at the back of the abdomen

Figure 11(b) Lymphangiogram showing dye outlining the lymph nodes (closed arrows). The open arrows show the kidney, ureters, and bladder outlined by an IVP (page 48)

into a lymph vessel and a similar procedure is carried out on the other foot. A dye that shows up on X-ray (a radio-opaque dye) is then slowly injected under slight pressure so that it fills the lymph vessels in the legs and abdomen (Figure 11). This part of the procedure is tedious and takes about 2 hours and it is a good idea for patients to take along a book or magazine. Occasional check films to follow the progress of the dye will be taken. Skin stitches will be put into the cut on the top of the foot at the end of the test once the needles have been removed. A dry dressing is put on the top of each foot.

- The test takes up to 4 hours and discomfort and tedium

- caused by lying still on the firm X-ray couch may be trouble-some.

- The blue-green dye is passed out in the urine which is green for some hours. Your complexion may become slightly greenish so that you look 'grey' and unwell. Some patients may have 'flu-like' symptoms.

- Occasional 'allergic reactions' to the blue-green dye or X-ray contrast dye may occur. If you feel breathless or faint, tell the doctor performing the test as the reaction can easiliy be reversed with simple drugs.

- Patients should sit with their legs raised as much as possible for the 24 hours after the test. This will stop swelling of the legs developing.

- Patients should not drive after this long examination as many will not feel up to it and driving may cause swelling of the feet.

- Try to avoid getting your feet wet for at least 24 hours, in order to avoid infection.

- *Day 2*. The next day a further series of X-rays of the abdomen and frequently an IVP (see page 35) will be done. Although there is usually no special preparation of the bowel, patients are often asked not to eat anything beforehand in order to get the best quality X-rays and IVP examination.

- This part of the test lasts about 1 hour.

- Many patients do not like driving after the IVP which often causes a temporary feeling of heat and flushing.

- The skin stitches in the feet should be removed 7–10 days after the test. A blue-green stain at the site of the injection on the top of the foot may persist for weeks and occasionally months.

- Soreness and swelling over the top of the foot are not uncommon and it is useful to have some pain-killing tablets available for the first few days after the test. Infection of the cut on the foot can occur and if the site of the stitches becomes very sore, inflamed, or discharges pus see your own doctor. There are no other long-term effects though the test will be avoided in patients whose lungs work poorly (such as in those with chronic bronchitis and emphysema) as some of the dye reaches the lungs and may *temporarily* reduce their ability to work normally.

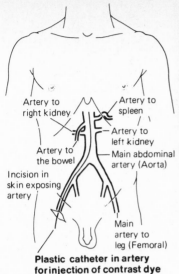

Artery to
right kidney

Artery to
spleen

Artery to
left kidney

Artery to
the bowel

Main abdominal
artery (Aorta)

Incision in
skin exposing
artery

Main
artery to
leg (Femoral)

**Plastic catheter in artery
for injection of contrast dye**

Figure 12(a) Diagrammatic representation of an arteriogram. In this case a plastic tube (catheter) has been introduced into the artery in the groin and fed up to the arteries in the abdomen. An X-ray dye is then injected to show up the blood vessels

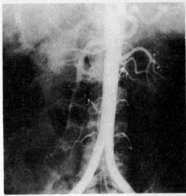

Figure 12(b) An arteriogram outlining these blood vessels

Arteriogram or venogram

These are tests used to outline an artery (arteriogram) or a vein (Figure 12). It is beyond the scope of this book to describe the techniques used for the different types of these tests as the method depends upon the site of the blood vessel being outlined.

● Briefly, it is necessary to place a fine plastic tube (a catheter) into the blood vessel being examined. This requires a minor operation which is usually done under local anaesthetic. If the test does require a general anaesthetic patients must not eat or drink for 6 hours before the anaesthetic. The technique needed to put the catheter into the blood vessel depends upon its site and should be discussed by the radiologist. In order to show up the vein or artery contrast dye is quickly injected and a rapid series of X-rays taken following it through the blood circulation of the area under investigation.

- During the injection of the dye patients feel hot and uncomfortable although this feeling goes away quickly.

- The length of time it takes depends on the blood vessel being investigated, though most tests should take less than 2 hours.

- Most patients will not want to drive after such a test. A small cut may be necessary to identify a blood vessel through which the catheter is passed. This cut may be at some distance. from the vessel being looked at as it is often not possible to get at the blood vessel directly. For instance it is common to use the blood vessels in the groin (femoral artery or vein) to get to blood vessels in the abdomen (Figure 12). If a cut is made the stitches will need to be removed about 7 days later.

- As with all tests using an injection of contrast dye, patients may very occasionally be allergic to the dye and if you become short of breath or feel faint you should tell the radiologist. Allergic reactions can easily be treated with simple drugs.

- There are usually no late complications though some bruising or discomfort where the catheter is put into the vein or artery is not uncommon. This should last only a few days.

Myelogram

A myelogram is an X-ray used to outline the *spinal canal* (the space around the spinal cord within the bony spine).

After injection of a local anaesthetic, a thin needle is passed between the bony vertebra in the lower back. The needle is then advanced into the fluid in the spinal canal (CSF). This initial part of the test is identical to a lumbar puncture and some fluid is usually withdrawn for laboratory tests. Contrast dye which shows up on an X-ray of the back can then be injected into the fluid in the spinal canal. If the patient is tipped this heavy dye flows down the canal to show if it is completely open the whole length of the spine. Any restriction (partial or complete) will show up. If an obstruction is complete (dye cannot flow past it) and the radiologist (usually a specialist in neurological X-rays) wants to show the length of the obstruction he may also put a needle into the spinal canal at the top of the spine. This allows dye to flow downwards to the restriction and will show the upper level of the blockage. Most myelograms do not require this extra procedure.

- This test should be relatively painless though there is some discomfort when the initial lumbar puncture is done.
- Special preparation is not required.
- The length of time needed for the tests depends partly on the findings, but this is usually less than 1 hour.
- Many patients having this test will be in-hospital patients and they will be asked to lie flat for some hours after the test to reduce the risk of headaches.
- There should be no long-term effects associated with the test. Some patients have a headache which will improve on lying flat.

Other specialized contrast tests

There are other special X-rays which are uncommon and beyond the scope of this book. Ask about such tests; the following points may be worth raising.

- What is the test for and how is it done?
- Is it uncomfortable?
- How long does it take?
- Are there any risks or side-effects?
- How will I feel after the test, can I go home, will I need someone to collect me; or will I be all right on my own?

44

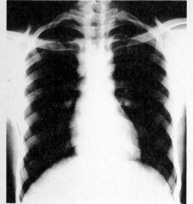

Figure 13(a) Chest X-ray which is relatively normal

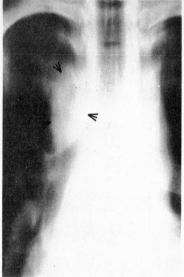

Figure 13(b) Close-up of a tomogram of the lungs of the same patient showing (see arrows) that the area around the heart (called the mediastinum) is wider than normal because of enlarged glands

Tomograms

Tomography is a special type of plain X-ray designed to get a better view of various parts of the body. When any X-ray is taken the image produced is made up of all the body's structures in front of the X-ray plate. In order to make unwanted structures blurred, whilst keeping the area being examined in focus, the X-ray machine used for tomography is swung in an arc over the patient. The image of structures in the plane in which the X-ray machine pivots stays in focus, whilst those in front or behind will be blurred. Small abnormalities (which may not be seen in an ordinary X-ray) can then be seen more clearly (Figure 13). A series of X-rays (known as cuts) of different parts of the area being examined are taken. After each cut the X-ray plate underneath the table will need to be changed.

The length of time the test takes will depend on the number of cuts required. A full test may take an hour and may sometimes be used with a contrast study.

- No special preparation is required.
- The test is, of course, painless and has no side-effects.
- Patients should be able to see themselves home afterwards.

ULTRASOUND (ULTRASONIC) TESTS

Rather than X-rays very high frequency sound waves are used for these tests. The frequency of the sound is far above that which the human ear can hear. A source of ultrasound waves is pressed against the body and a beam of sound waves is sent into the body. These waves strike areas of different density and sound waves are bounced back rather like the ASDIC system used to detect submarines (Figure 14).

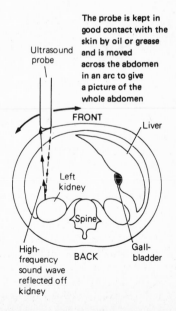

Figure 14 How ultrasound works (see text for explanation)

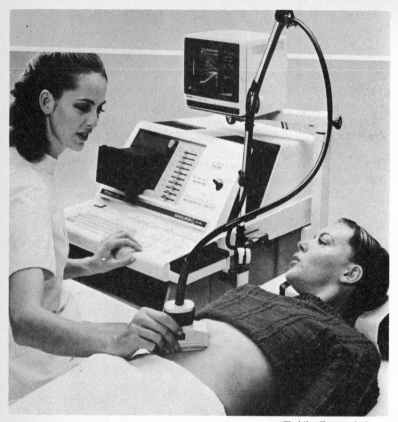

(*Toshiba Corporation*)

Figure 15 A patient having an ultrasound test

- When the test is done a probe looking rather like a micro-phone is used. This must be in good contact with the skin and the skin is coated with oil or grease. The probe is moved in an arc over the skin and sends out and detects the reflected sound; the information is used to build up a picture of the area being examined (Figure 15). This is displayed on a television screen, and when the picture is complete an instant (polaroid) picture is taken for a permanent record.

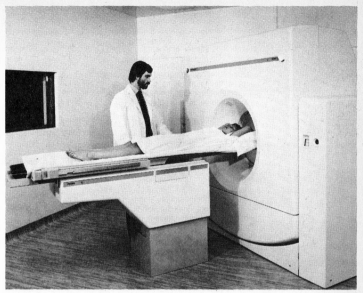

(*Philips Medical Systems*)

Figure 16 A patient about to have a CT scan. The patient will be moved into the centre of the machine as X-rays are taken of the chest and abdomen

- No special preparation is required. However, if the gall-bladder (page 36) is to be examined, patients will be asked not to eat anything for 6 hours beforehand, and if the lower abdomen or pelvis is to be shown, patients will be asked to come for the test with a **full** bladder.
- The test is entirely painless and ultrasound has no side-effects.
- Patients will suffer no effects from the test and may drive immediately.

CT BODY SCAN (also known as CAT scan, whole body scan, or a body scanner)

This is a revolutionary new method of taking X-rays. It differs from a normal X-ray in two ways. First there is no normal X-ray film; instead there is an electronic X-ray detector. The second major difference is that both the X-ray source (equivalent to the old X-ray machine) and the detector rotate around the patient (Figure 16). The X-ray scanner produces a narrow beam of X-rays and as this rotates around the part of the body being examined, the detector receives information on the density or consistency of the body at that point. When the scanner and detector have finished rotating around the body, the information from all angles is processed by a computer which produces a picture showing the density of all the body's structures in the area about which it has rotated. The picture is equivalent to a 'slice' through the body as the beam is narrow (about 1 cm) (Figure 16). The slice shows the different parts of the body clearly as their densities vary. A full examination of the body requires numerous slices so that a three-dimensional picture can be built up. A photographic record of each slice is available and a more detailed computerized picture can be printed.

- CT scans are not used for routine X-rays as they are expensive and take longer than a normal plain X-ray which is perfectly adequate for most everyday uses. However, when careful examination of small or indistinct structures is required, then the CT scan is often the most accurate method. It will not replace many of the special X-ray studies previously discussed, but will be used together with other techniques.

- CT scans of the abdomen are usually done after preparation of the bowel. This requires the administration of a laxative for 2 days before the test.

- During the test it may be necessary for the patient to drink a rather unpleasant tasting liquid which outlines the stomach and bowel. During CT scan examinations of the brain, injections of dye may be given to see a possible abnormality will absorb the dye and this injection may cause a temporary feeling of heat or discomfort.

- The duration of a test depends on the extent of the examination but several X-ray slices will be needed so that the test often takes about 1 hour.

- CT scans are painless though sick patients may find them tedious and some patients dislike the dye they may be asked to drink. Injections of contrast dye may be uncomfortable for a short while.

- Most patients are able to see themselves home after a CT scan, but many would prefer some help.

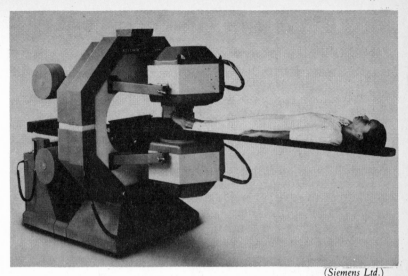

(*Siemens Ltd.*)

Figure 17 A patient about to have an isotope scan. The gamma camera detects the amount of radioactivity in the body and produces a picture

RADIO ISOTOPE TESTS (isotope imaging or scans)

These tests use injections or very small amounts of radioactive substances which are absorbed by various parts of the body and show up on special photographs taken with a radiation scanner (Figure 17). These tests rely on the radioactive substance, or *isotope*, being taken up preferentially by the part of the body being examined. Different isotopes are therefore selected for examination of various parts of the body.

Bone scan

A radioactive isotope is used that accumulates in parts of bone that are actively making new bone. Because of this the picture formed is different from an X-ray as the areas of greatest accumulation of isotope are at sites of bone activity. Increased bone activity (hot areas) may be due to repair of damage (a fracture or arthritis), as well as tumour. Some tumours do not take up the isotope and appear as areas of decreased uptake (cold areas).

- No special preparation is required.
- A painless injection of the isotope is given into a vein in the arm.
- The scan or imaging is done about 2 hours later. The patient lies on a firm couch while a radioactive detector or camera produces a picture.
- Patients will be able to drive immediately after the test ends, which should be less than 3 hours from the injection.

Liver scan

The isotope used for this test is taken up by the liver, and areas of the liver that are not working normally will show as a 'hole' or 'cold area'.

- No special preparation is required.
- A painless injection of isotope is given into an arm vein.
- The scan is done about 20 minutes later and will take about half an hour.
- Patients are able to drive immediately after the test.
- The test takes about 1 hour.

Gall-bladder and biliary scans

This test is used to outline the gall-bladder (which contains bile) and the ducts connecting it to the liver and bowel. The test should not be done for at least one week after a barium meal (page 30).

- No special preparation is necessary.
- A painless injection of isotope is given into a vein in an arm.
- Images or scans of the liver are taken immediately and after several hours. Occasionally a further scan may be done at 24 hours.
- Patients can go home afterwards and are fit to drive.
- The length of time the test takes is variable and depends on how quickly the isotope gets into the gall-bladder. Most tests

take less than 4 hours though some patients may need to return for a further scan the next day.

Lung scans

Lung scans can be used to show two things, (a) the blood flow (perfusion) through the lungs, and (b) the flow of air into the lungs (ventilation). Because of this two different isotopes may be used.

- No special preparation is necessary.
- A painless injection of isotope is given into an arm vein (perfusion scan).
- Patients may also be asked to breathe in an isotope (a gas) through an oxygen mask (ventilation).
- Scans of the lungs are taken immediately.
- Patients are able to make their own way home.
- The test should take less than 1 hour.

Thryoid scans

The isotope used for these scans is taken up by the thyroid so that an overactive area shows up as a 'hot spot' and an inactive one as a hole or 'cold area'.

- Patients will be given a list of drugs to avoid before the test. These include iodine, antithyroid drugs, thyroid replacement therapy, and some of the contrast radiological dyes used for special X-rays (page 30). Patients who have not been given a list, or are in doubt of which drugs or medicines are permissible, should ask the doctor who is to perform the test.

- No other special preparation is needed.
- A painless injection of isotope is given in a vein in the arm.
- Scans of the thyroid are done about 20 minutes later.
- Occasionally patients will be given a dose of isotope by mouth and be asked to return for a scan 24 hours later.
- Patients feel well enough to go home immediately.
- The test should take less than 1 hour.

Kidney (renal) scans

The isotope used is excreted by the kidneys and tests the function of the kidneys.

- No special preparation is required though the test is best done before an IVP (see page 34). If an IVP has been done a gap of 3 days should be left before the scan.
- A painless injection of isotope is given into an arm vein.
- Scanning may begin immediately or may be delayed for 1 hour depending on the information required.
- Patients are able to go home unaccompanied after the test.
- The test should take less than 2 hours.

Other isotope scans

There are other specialized isotope scans which are used occasionally to investigate cancer patients. If you are to have such a scan, discuss the test with your doctor and ask the questions suggested at the end of this section. Nearly all isotope scans are painless and cause little inconvenience.

SPECIAL BIOPSIES

A biopsy, the removal of some tissue to examine under the microscope, may be done to make the diagnosis of cancer or to see if a cancer has spread to other tissues. Many tissues can be biopsied and some of the common types of biopsy are discussed below. All biopsies carry a small risk of complications, such as infection or bruising, and it is important to discuss these with the doctor before the test is done.

Lymph node biopsy

Lymph nodes are the glands that respond to infection, they may, for instance, be felt in the neck as painful lumps when a child has tonsillitis. These glands are not confined to the neck but are scattered throughout the body. They are particularly concentrated in the neck, around the collar bones, under the arms, around the major blood vessels in the abdomen, around the heart, and in the groins. In many of these places the lymph nodes are just under the skin so that glands can be felt and if necessary removed surgically — biopsied. The type of surgery and anaesthetic, local or general, will depend on the size and location of the lymph node. Many of these operations are simple and can be done as a day patient. As a cut must be made in a skin, stitches will be put in and will need to be removed about a week later. Occasionally it may be possible to remove a small portion of a lymph node using a needle — a needle biopsy. No anaesthetic or formal operation is then required, though the small size and condition of the tissue may make it more difficult to make a diagnosis when it is examined with a microscope. Patients will need to discuss the need for, the methods to be used and the side-effects of any biopsy. Following a biopsy the tissue must be prepared before it is examined, and a result will not be available for 24 or more hours. Occasionally sophisticated tests may take several days.

Bone marrow biopsy and aspirate

The *bone marrow* (elements within the bone that form blood) may be sampled to see if it is involved with a cancer or to test the effects of chemotherapy or radiotherapy (discussed later) on its ability to form new blood cells.

- A bone marrow aspirate is done with a small needle which is used to suck some particles from the bone. The test is usually done by locally anaesthetizing or freezing the skin over the breast bone (sternum) or a pelvic bone and then inserting a short needle into the bone. With good local anaesthesia this is not uncomfortable, though there is usually momentary pain when the syringe is used to suck a little of the marrow substance out. The test is done in a few minutes and there should be no side-effects, apart from slight local bruising. The results can be available within a few hours.

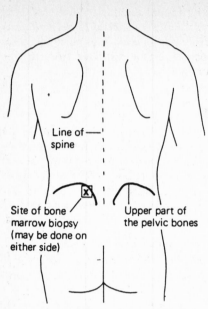

Line of — spine

X

Site of bone marrow biopsy (may be done on either side)

Upper part of the pelvic bones

Figure 18 Diagrammatic representation of the usual site for a bone marrow biopsy

- A bone marrow biopsy or trephine is usually done together with an aspirate, but because it means removing a small piece of the bone marrow it is not done from the breast bone as this is too thin. Instead it is usually taken from the prominent pelvic bones over the lower back (Figure 18). It may also be taken from the pelvic bones forming the border to the front of the abdomen or pelvis. Local anaesthetic is injected to deaden pain though some patients may also require a pre-medication with a tranquillizer or a pain killer if they are particularly anxious or sensitive to pain. A thin needle is then inserted through the anaesthetized skin into the bone, and is used to remove a small core of bone. This part of the test may be uncomfortable as the local anaesthetic may not deaden *all* the pain from the bone itself. The test should take only a few minutes and many patients do not require extra pain killers. The pain only lasts a short while and there are no long-term side-effects of the biopsy.

- Most patients should be able to drive after the test — provided they have not had tranquillizers or pain killers.
- The test may take several days to interpret as the calcium (the bony part) must be dissolved from the biopsy before it can be examined.

Liver biopsy

Small pieces of tissue may be taken from the liver for examination under a microscope in a variety of conditions, malignant and non-malignant. Liver biopsy requires a short stay in hospital. Before the biopsy is done your blood should be examined to ensure that it will clot normally. There may very rarely be some internal bleeding after a biopsy and blood is usually cross-matched in case a transfusion should be required.

- The skin overlying the site of the biopsy (on the right side of the abdomen) is anaesthetized with local anaesthetic. A small cut may then be made so that it is easier to insert the biopsy needle.
- The doctor doing the test will explain how he wants you to breathe as it is important that the chest and liver are still at the moment of biopsy. You will be asked to take a deep breath and to breath out deeply and hold your breath till the biopsy is done.
- When you and the doctor are happy that this can done a thin needle is introduced through the anaesthetized skin till it is just over the liver. When you have breathed out and the liver is still (it normally moves up and down with each breath) the needle is pushed quickly into and then pulled out of the liver. A syringe is attached to the needle and suction is applied during this movement so that a small piece of liver is sucked into the needle and removed from the liver. There is usually a momentary feeling of pain at this stage of the test which is all over very quickly.
- You will then be left to rest quietly and your pulse and blood pressure will be recorded regularly for a number of hours. This is to make sure that there has been no internal bleeding from the liver surface. If you feel pain in the abdomen or over the right shoulder, call the nurse or doctor. Irritation of the right side of the diaphragm (muscular wall between

the abdomen and chest) often causes pain in the tip of the right shoulder and this may happen without abdominal pain.

- Provided that you feel well and your pulse and blood pressure are normal (as in the vast majority) you can go home later, though this will depend on the attitude of your local hospital. Some doctors will do liver biopsies as a day procedure whilst others may ask patients to stay in overnight. The test itself should take less than half an hour.
- There should be little discomfort during the procedure, apart from a jab of pain at the moment of the biopsy. Side-effects are uncommon; if bleeding occurs a blood transfusion may be needed and if it continues an operation may rarely be required. Leakage of bile from the liver is another rare complication that may need to be corrected by operation. It must be stressed that such complications are very unusual, but it is useful to discuss the procedure and its potential complications with the doctor performing the test.
- Some patients do not feel particularly well afterwards so it is best to arrange for someone to accompany you home.
- Tissue from the biopsy is usually ready to be examined within 1–2 days.

Pleural biopsy and aspirate

If fluid collects in the space between the lung and chest wall (the pleural space) a biopsy of the lining of the chest wall (the pleura) may be done to determine the cause — usually infection or tumour. In this situation fluid is often drained off the chest (aspirated) regardless of whether a pleural biopsy is done.

- A local anaesthetic is injected into the skin of the chest wall between the ribs and often a small cut is made in the skin so that the needle can enter easily. When the chest wall is 'frozen' a short needle is pushed through the small cut into the fluid in the chest. If fluid only is to be removed the needle is attached to a syringe or small suction bottle and the fluid withdrawn. If a pleural biopsy is to be done a small piece of the pleura is cut out in a small notch in the needle. The rest of the fluid may then be removed.
- The moment of the biopsy may be uncomfortable though this should be minimized by a good injection of local anaesthetic.

- If you experience chest pain, shortness of breath, or a desire to cough, tell the doctor. If fluid is removed too quickly the shift position of the lungs may cause these symptoms which are a sign to stop or abandon the procedure. Most patients feel some of these sensations at the end of the test when the last of the fluid is being removed.

- One complication of the test is a build-up of air in the pleural space between the chest wall and lung (a *pneumothorax*). This may happen if some air gets in by the needle or if the needle scratches the lung surface and causes leakage of air from the lung. Because of this risk a chest X-ray should be performed after the test to check if there has been an air leak. Small amounts of air in the pleural space are not important and can be watched, but large amounts of air will cause collapse of the lung on that side. This complication is unusual, but may mean that a plastic tube must be inserted into the chest to suck out the air. This usually needs to be left in for several days to ensure that the lung re-expands.

- The test can often be done as a day procedure, though if the lung collapses because of air in the pleural space it will be necessary for the patient to stay in hospital. The test itself takes less than half an hour.

- For those who can go home afterwards it would be best to arrange for someone to collect them.

- Fluid from the chest is sent for examination under a microscope (cytology) as well as the biopsy of the pleura.

Skin biopsy

Biopsy of abnormal areas of the skin are frequently taken to determine whether they are cancerous or not. Very small biopsies may be taken with a special punch, or a larger biopsy may be taken. A punch biopsy only takes a few seconds and is relatively painless. A larger biopsy will require the cutting out of a piece of skin and then stitching the small wound togetherl. Under a good local anaesthetic the procedure should be painless.

- There should be no side-effects.
- The stitches will need to be removed between 5 and 10 days afterwards, depending on where the biopsy is.

- You should be able to drive after a skin biopsy, provided no sedative has been given.

BLOOD TESTS

The taking of blood (venepuncture) is the commonest type of test in medicine. Blood is taken from a vein in the arm and is used for a wide variety of tests.

- A tight elastic cuff (torniquet) is put around the upper arm. This slows the blood flow in the veins draining the arm and the veins on the surface stand out because of this.
- When the skin on the arm has been cleaned with a special swab a needle is pushed into the vein and blood sucked into a syringe. Blood is usually taken from the veins in the inside of the elbow though other veins over the back of the arm, hand, or inside of the forearm may be used. Although not normally needed, quite large quantities of blood (100–200 ml) may be taken without *any* side-effects.
- No local anaesthetic is needed and there should be very little discomfort when blood is taken skilfully. Occasionally veins may be difficult and more than one attempt may be necessary. One of the main reasons for failure to get blood is inadequate dilatation (filling) of the veins. If despite a torniquet the veins do not stand out it may be worth putting your arm in hot water to increase the blood flow. Some patients who have had chemotherapy (drug treatment, Chapter 12) given by injection may have very difficult veins as the drugs often cause clotting and damage to the veins. In such cases blood should only be taken by those used to dealing with these cases.
- After the blood has been taken the needle is removed and a cotton-wool swab is pressed firmly over the needle puncture for a few minutes to prevent bleeding.
- There should be no side-effects apart from a little local bruising.
- Very occasionally patients feel faint when having their blood taken and it is best not to watch the nurse or doctor doing it. The vast majority will be able to leave immediately and can see themselves home.

LARYNGOSCOPY

This is the examination of the voice box (larynx). A mirror is used for the test.

- A mirror is warmed up (to prevent breath condensing on it).
- You are asked to poke your tongue out.
- The tip of the tongue is held by the doctor using some gauze.
- The doctor then puts the mirror (like a dentist's) into the back of your mouth.
- Using a head mirror or light source he looks down your throat at the larynx.

The test is only mildly uncomfortable if done expertly and takes a few minutes.

CERVICAL SMEAR

As there are rarely early signs or symptoms of *cervical cancer* (cancer of the cervix or neck of the womb, page 141) it has become normal to examine the surface of the cervix when a pelvic examination if done. This should be done periodically when screening for cervical cancer.

- During the pelvic examination the walls of the vagina are held apart with an instrument called a speculum, so that the cervix can be seen. A wooden spatula is then scraped over the surface of the cervix and the cells on the spatula are then smeared on a glass slide. After the cells have been stained they are examined under a microscope to check if there are any early signs of cancer.
- The examination should be only slightly uncomfortable.
- No special preparation is required and there are no side-effects after the test.
- Results of the test can be ready in a day or so.

DIRECT VISUAL EXAMINATIONS INSIDE THE BODY (endoscopy)

Sigmoidoscopy

Sigmoidoscopy is an examination of the rectum and last part of the large bowel (Figure 19). A lubricated stainless steel tube

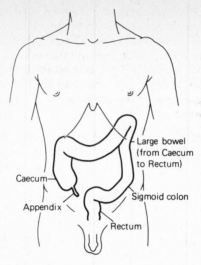

Figure 19 Diagrammatic representation of the course of the large bowel

is passed gently into the back passage (rectum). This has a light inside so that the operator can see into the rectum. It is connected to a hand-operated bulb which pumps air at low pressure into the rectum and expands the large bowel. As the bowel is expanded the sigmoidoscope (the tube in the rectum) can be pushed further into the large bowel. Using this instrument it is possible to examine up to 18 cm of the last part of the large bowel. As most cancers develop in this area, it is an important examination. It is possible, using a wire snare or swab, to remove small polyps from the bowel for microscopic examination.

- Apart from mild discomfort the test is painless.
- No preparation is required though the test cannot be done if the rectum is loaded with faeces.
- There are no side-effects and patients are able to leave immediately and to drive.

Colonoscopy

This is a method for looking further into the large bowel using an instrument called a colonoscope. A sigmoidoscope is a straight metal tube and it can only be used to examine the last part of the large bowel (rectum and sigmoid colon). A colonoscope is made from optical fibres which can be bent and the instrument can be guided around curves so that the whole of the large bowel (Figure 19) can be examined. The colonoscopy transmits a bright light and allows to doctor to look into the bowel. As light follows the curve of the fibres it is possible to see round corners.

- Preparation of the bowel is necessary and you will be given instructions to take laxatives for two days before the test. An enema may be used prior to the test to ensure that the bowel is empty.
- The test is usually done as an out-patient, though may hospitals admit patients to a day ward.
- A sedative may be given prior to the test.
- The lubricated colonoscope is then passed into the rectum whilst you lie curled up on your side.
- The instrument is gradually advanced in the large bowel and the inside of the bowel examined on the way and photographs can be taken if required.
- It is usually possible to examine the whole of the large bowel and to biopsy (page 52) any polyps on the way. A snare is used to remove the polyp, often with a hook being used to hold it. This should not be unduly uncomfortable.
- The test is finished when the colonscopy is removed. There may be some discomfort with the investigation, but this should not be severe.
- Patients can leave immediately after the test but should arrange for a taxi or someone to collect them and should not drive after a sedative.

Gastroscopy

This is the use of a flexible instrument to look into the gullet (oesophagus), stomach, and upper bowel (duedenum) (see Figure 20). The gastroscope is made from optical fibres which can be bent. The doctor performing the investigation is able to guide the gastroscope so that he can look around the stomach.
- You will be asked not to eat or drink from the night before the test. This is to ensure that there is no food in the stomach.

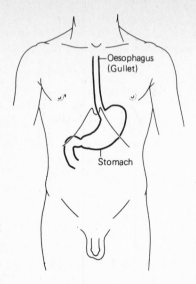

Figure 20 Diagrammatic representation of the upper gastrointestinal tract

- The test is usually done as an out-patient, though many hospitals admit their patients to a day ward.
- A sedative is given before the test: this is often an injection into a vein which will make you sleepy, reduces discomfort, and means that you often remember little of the actual test. Local anaesthetic is also sprayed into the back of the throat to reduce discomfort and a tendency to gag.
- When preparations are complete the lubricated end of the gastroscope is guided into your mouth and throat so that it is swallowed into the gullet or oesophagus. The gullet is examined visually as the instrument is passed into the stomach. Photographs may be taken at any part of the test.
- As the gastroscope is passed further it comes into the stomach. The doctor can then manoeuvre the tip of the instrument to examine all parts of the stomach.
- The tip can also be guided into the last part of the stomach as it becomes the duodenum. This area between the duedenum and stomach is a common site of ulcers. The gastroscope can be passed through into the duodenum and the

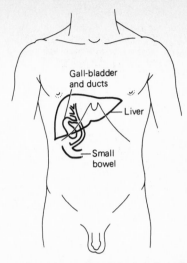

Figure 21 Diagrammatic representation of the duct from the gall-bladder to the small bowel; the pancreatic duct joins the bowel in the same place and both may be examined during an ERCP

entrance of the bile duct and duct from the pancreas can be examined. In addition to examining, and photographing any suspicious areas, biopsies (page 52) may be taken. This should not cause any discomfort.

- When the test is completed the gastroscope is taken out.
- Because a strong sedative has been used you will need to rest and recover from the test.
- You should not drive after the test as you have had a sedative injection.
- The test will take about 1 hour but with time to recover from the sedative you should expect to be at the hospital for most of the day.

ERCP (examination of the ducts to the gall-bladder and pancreas)

ERCP (standing for, in medical language, endoscopic retrograde cholangiopancreatography) is a test using a gastroscope (see

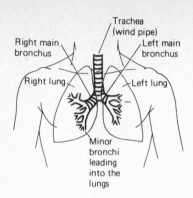

Figure 22 Diagrammatic representation of the main airways leading into the lungs. These can be examined through a bronchoscope

above) to examine and inject X-ray contrast dye into the ducts from the gall-bladder and pancreas, as they enter the duodenum (Figure 21).

- A gastroscopy is carried out. This requires the preparation described in the previous section.
- When the gastroscope is in the duodenum the tiny entrances of the ducts are identified. They usually enter the bowel through a small raised area known as the ampulla of Vater. A fine plastic tube (catheter) is passed down the gastroscope and into the opening of the duct. The doctor can select either the bile duct or the pancreatic duct. The test is difficult and requires a skilled gastroscopist. When the catheter is in the duct a small amount of X-ray dye is injected and a series of X-rays taken.
- The test itself may take about 1 hour.
- Recovery time is required after the sedative.
- Patients should *not* attempt to drive home and will need to be collected.
- The test is usually done as an out-patient though admission to a day ward is common.

Bronchoscopy

Bronchoscopy is a test during which a doctor looks directly into the main airways into the lung (bronchi) (Figure 22). In the past rigid metal bronchoscopes were used but the introduction of flexible fibre-optic bronchoscopes has made the test much easier. The optical fibres in these bronchoscopes can be bent and transmit light into the chest and allow the doctor to see into the main airways.

- The test can be done as an out-patient though patients may be admitted to hospital.
- Sedation is usually given before the test.
- The back of the throat is sprayed with a local anaesthetic to reduce discomfort and the tendency to gag.
- The flexible bronchoscope is thin and is passed into the back of the throat through a nostril.
- Photographs can be taken during the examination and pieces of tumour (biopsies) taken for examination.

QUESTIONS TO ASK ABOUT INVESTIGATIONS

If further information on the tests described or other more specialized investigations not discussed is required, these questions may be useful.

(1) Why is the test necessary?
(2) How is the test done?
(3) Is any preparation needed?
(4) Is the test uncomfortable or unpleasant?
(5) Are there any immediate side-effects?
(6) How long does the test take?
(7) Are there any long-term side-effects?
(8) Will I need to be admitted to hospital for the test?
(9) If not, can I go home on my own and am I safe to drive?

CHAPTER 10

Surgery for cancer

Surgery was the first effective treatment of cancer and it is still the main treatment for most localized tumours. During this century more complicated surgery has become routine because of improved surgical techniques and anaesthetic and post-operative care.

Surgery is important: it cures more patients of cancer than radiotherapy and drug therapy together.

DIAGNOSIS

Before a diagnosis of cancer can be made a biopsy **MUST** be taken. A biopsy (page 52) is the surgical removal of a sample of tissue, such as a lymph node, for examination under a microscope. Biopsies are usually performed by surgeons though some of the tests may be done by other doctors. They are frequently done under local anaesthetic or as a day procedure. Most biopsies do not turn out to show cancer and biopsies may be taken to look for other diseases.

There are several ways to obtain a sample of tissue. The method used will depend on where the lump is and the size of the biopsy needed. Common types of biopsy are listed below and are described more fully in Chapter 9.

- Excision biopsy. This is the surgical removal of the whole tumour. This is frequently done for small tumours of the breast and skin cancers. If a lump can be removed in one piece this is ideal.
- Incisional biopsy. Only part of the lump is removed during this procedure. It is usually done when the lump is too large to be removed easily.
- Needle biopsy. A needle is inserted into a lump and part of the tissue or fluid within the tumour is cut or sucked out.
- Endoscopic biopsy. When a tube is passed into the body to see areas that are not normally visible the technique is known

as endoscopy (page 59). Biopsies of small pieces of tissue may be taken using the tube or endoscope. The common types of tests are:

(a) Gastroscopy and oesophagoscopy, examination of the gullet, stomach, and first part of bowel (page 61).
(b) Sigmoidoscopy, examination of rectum and last part of bowel (page 59).
(c) Colonoscopy, examination of the large bowel (page 60).
(d) Bronchoscopy, examination of the air passages into the lungs (page 64).
(e) Cystoscopy, examination of the urinary bladder.
(f) Laryngoscopy, examination of the throat and voice box.
(g) Colposcopy, examination of the cervix (neck of the womb) and vaginal examination.

STAGING (see Chapters 8 and 9)

Although most staging is done by special X-rays and other tests surgeons are asked to help to stage certain types of tumour. In Hodgkin's disease, for instance, (page 179) staging may include examination and removal of the spleen and lymph nodes within the abdomen. This operation is called a staging laparotomy. Such operations for staging are only done in a few special cancers and most surgical staging procedures consist of needle biopsies or endoscopy. Staging is often crucial for the choice of treatment and surgical examination and removal of tissue may be the most accurate way of finding how much a cancer has spread.

CURATIVE SURGERY FOR LOCALIZED CANCER

It a tumour has not spread to distant parts of the body then it is potentially curable with surgery or radiotherapy. It is crucial that all the cancerous tissue is removed, or the tumour will recur.

It is therefore essential that all tumour that can be seen together with a wide margin of normal tissue is removed. Although such an operation can be mutilating the choice may be between disfigurement or a spreading tumour which could end in death.

Surgeons will often attempt to remove nearby lymph nodes. If these are taken with the original tumour in one piece the operation is called *en bloc* resection. More distant draining lymph nodes may also be removed in the case of certain tumours. This is because the surgeon knows that the risk of spread is high, even though they may not appear abnormal.

SURGERY TO CONTROL SYMPTOMS

Operations designed to control or prevent symptoms but not to cure are called 'palliative'. No attempt is made to remove all the tumour; the operation is designed to deal with specific problems. If, for instance, the bowel is obstructed by a tumour that cannot be removed, the surgeon can by-pass the obstruction so that pain caused by the obstruction is relieved. The pain and effects of the operation must be balanced against the possible gains and the patient's life expectancy. Careful thought is required before palliative surgery, but it can be of great benefit to patients and can prolong life.

SURGERY TO PREVENT CANCER

The removal of growths that may, if left, turn into cancers is commonly forgotten, but is important in certain tumours. Perhaps the commonest operation is the removal of polyps from the colon. Rarely, drastic operations such as removal of the colon for familial polyposis (page 4) or chronic ulcerative colitis (page 5) are needed when the risk of cancer is very high.

SIDE-EFFECTS

All operations are likely to cause some discomfort and carry a risk of complications. It is worth asking your doctor about any risks of the particular operation you may undergo.

Questions to ask before an operation

(1) General questions

Why is this operation being chosen, and what exactly will be done?

Are there any other ways of dealing with the problem besides surgery?
What is the usual stay in hospital and how long before I am really fit?
How much pain will there be and are there any risks?
What about cigarettes — are they dangerous, should I give them up before coming into hospital?
Where will the scar be, will it be obvious?
Will there be any other treatment afterwards?

(2) Biopsy

How will the biopsy be done?
Will an anaesthetic be necessary?
If the biopsy shows cancer, will the surgeon carry on to a full operation at the same time?
Is it necessary to stay in hospital overnight after the biopsy?
Should I arrange transport or can I see myself home?
Are there any side-effects?

(3) Curative surgery

Why is the operation being done?
Are there any other alternatives to an operation?
Is there any special preparation necessary?
How long will I have to stay afterwards?
Is the operation uncomfortable and are there any possible side-effects?
Does anyone ever die from the operation?
Where will the scar be and is it disfiguring?
Is any special appliance needed afterwards, such as a colostomy?
Will any further operation be needed?
Is any other treatment planned?

The surgeons may not be able to give a definite answer to all of these questions before an operation, as the exact procedure will depend on the stage of the cancer found at the operation, but should be able to give an idea of what to expect.

(4) Palliative surgery (to prevent symptoms)

How much will the operation help or prevent symptoms?

How much pain is caused by the operation?
Will the operation have other unwanted effects?
Does anyone ever die from the operation?
How long will I be in hospital?
Are there other ways of treating or preventing the symptoms?

CHAPTER 11

Radiotherapy for cancer

Radiotherapy (also called radiation therapy, deep X-ray therapy, cobalt treatment, or irradiation) is the use of high energy rays to kill cancer cells. Most radiotherapy is given by a machine some distance away from the patient (external therapy) though small amounts of radioactive material (implants) may be placed inside the body for a few days during internal therapy.

Radiation damages the ability of cells to divide and multiply; this affects both normal and cancer cells and all cells are sensitive to irradiation if a high enough dose is given. The dose of radiotherapy that can be given safely depends on the effect of the irradiation on the normal tissues. A dose that does not cause severe side-effects is used and this will often kill cancer cells within a tumour and reduce its size or destroy it completely. Radiotherapy works in some tumours because they are more easily damaged than normal tissues.

Radiotherapy can be used in a variety of ways. It may totally destroy a tumour and cure the patient. In other situations where a tumour is too large to be removed, radiotherapy is sometimes used to shrink the cancer so that it can be surgically removed. It may also be used together with drug treatment (chemotherapy) to get the best response in certain cancers. It is particularly useful in reducing a wide variety of symptoms, including pain.

In recent times there have been important improvements in radiotherapy. Modern machines can deliver more radiation to a cancer whilst giving a smaller dose to the surrounding normal tissues and skin. Other major improvements have come from a better understanding of the normal behaviour of cancers by doctors using radiotherapy (radiotherapists).

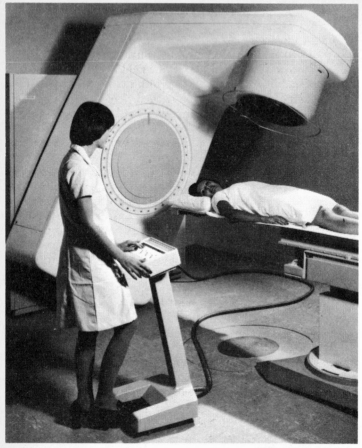

(Philips Medical Systems)

Figure 23 Modern radiotherapy machine (a linear accelerator)

HOW IS RADIOTHERAPY GIVEN?

- The first visit to a radiotherapy department usually does not involve treatment. A radiotherapist will tell you about the treatment and make an examination prior to starting treatment. There may well be further X-rays or other tests to define the site of the cancer and treatment is then 'planned'. During planning, the area (field or portal) to be treated is marked out on the skin. A purple dye (which must not be washed off) may be used or some small tattoos (dots, only) are used to outline the corners of the field. After this has been done the radiotherapist will work with a radiation physicist to calculate the dose of radiation needed. This will depend on the type of cancer, the site involved, and the person's body shape.

- Treatment usually consists of a series of individual treatments which are called fractions. The number of fractions needed will again depend on several factors. Treatment may be almost daily (Monday–Friday) for around 2–4 weeks. If you are about to receive radiotherapy ask how often the treatment is given and how long it is to continue (remembering that the plan may need to be changed). The treatment is split into fractions in order to protect the normal tissues; it is usually more effective to give small doses of radiotherapy each day than to give one large dose.

- What are the machines like? Although there are different types of radiotherapy machines, most people's immediate reaction is of 'how enormous and complex they are' (Figure 23). Not only are they big but the machine or table that the patient lies on may move up or down or rotate, often with a humming noise. The whole complicated machine and its array of controls is designed to give a carefully designed dose of radiotherapy with safety. It is normal for anyone to feel frightened by the machinery but most patients quickly become used to it.

- The treatment is given by a radiographer specially trained in giving radiotherapy. Using the tattoos or painted markers they will position the person on the table for treatment. Parts of the body may be protected by lead blocks placed above or on the body. For certain tumours a plastic shield may be used to hold the patient still during treatment. This is particularly common during radiation therapy to the head when it is important to make sure the area treated is exactly the same each time. Plastic shields or moulds are often specially made for individual patients and special measurements may be taken before treatment can start.

- The radiographer will not stay in the room during treatment.

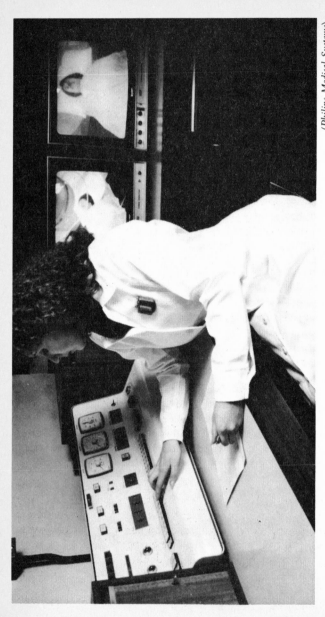

(Philips Medical Systems)

Figure 24 A radiographer controlling radiotherapy treatment. The patient can
be seen on a television screen behind the radiographer and she can talk to him
through an intercom

She will be in another room and will be able to see the patient on a TV screen or through a thick window and can talk to them through a loudspeaker system (Figure 24). Patients are watched throughout the treatment, which usually only takes a few minutes.

- Various types of equipment may be used according to the cancer. Orthovoltage radiotherapy machines (of relatively low energy) were one of the first type of equipment used to treat cancer. Their main disadvantages are an inability to penetrate skin well and difficulty in focusing the beam so that surrounding normal tissue is treated as well. Because, in the past, doctors tried to use it to give high doses to internal tumours, it sometimes caused skin burns giving radiotherapy a bad name. Cobalt and linear accelerators are more modern machines that give high doses to the tumour and less to the skin. They can be better focused and the dose to surrounding tissues is low. Most cancers are now treated on one or other of these machines. Other machines using different types of radition are experimental at present.

No one is radioactive from treatment and they are not a risk to other people.

SIDE-EFFECTS OF RADIOTHERAPY

As radiation effects both normal and cancer cells it is not surprising that it causes side-effects. Not everyone gets side-effects, though. Their type and their severity depend on the part of the body being treated, the dose of radiotherapy, the way it is split up into fractions, and other drug treatment (especially anticancer drugs) that may be given at the same time.

- The most common side-effect of radiation is tiredness. This may build up during treatment but will improve in the first few weeks after stopping treatment. Along with tiredness many patients lose their appetite and some feel sick. Advice on eating during therapy is given on page 269.
- Many patients notice slight reddening of the skin, like sunburn, and tanning of the treated skin is common at the end of the radiotherapy. This is expected and will clear up by itself. If, as occasionally happens, the skin starts to break

down and weep, tell your radiotherapist or radiographer. It is important to take care of the skin being treated so avoid using soaps, perfumes, cosmetics, hot-water bottles, and UV or heat lamps on the area being treated. Ointments should not be put on the area without asking the radiotherapist's advice and the area should be protected from sunlight or extreme cold. Patients who need to shave should use an electric razor if the skin of the face is being treated.

- Diarrhoea. When the abdomen is being treated, diarrhoea may be a problem. Tell your radiotherapist if this is a problem; he may prescribe specific treatment. The following suggestions may be helpful for controlling the symptoms. See if a clear liquid diet will allow the diarrhoea to settle. Avoid foods that may cause cramping — these include spirits, spicy foods, coffee, cabbage, cauliflower, broccoli, and baked beans. If a liquid diet does not get rid of the diarrhoea small amounts of food should be eaten frequently and plenty of fluids drunk. Milk products are usually not helpful and should be avoided. As the diarrhoea improves, soft low fibre foods should be added into the diet.

- Radiotherapy to the head and neck may cause particular side-effects. A sore throat on swallowing or eating can be troublesome. If this is the case change your diet to soft, well cooked foods. All solids should be cut up into small bites and moistened with gravy; spicy foods and spirits should be avoided. If necessary, the diet should be supplemented with liquid high calorie and protein drinks such as Complan (page 270). Your radiotherapists may prescribe a liquid local anaesthetic that should be drunk before eating so that pain on swallowing is reduced.

- If the radiotherapy area includes the mouth, take special care of your teeth. Patients with bad teeth should preferably see their dentist before treatment and tell him that they are going to receive radiotherapy. Teeth should be cleaned regularly (up to 4 times a day) with a soft round bristle brush and a smooth fluoride toothpaste used. After cleaning your teeth, rinse out your mouth with a solution of salt and baking soda (1 teaspoon of each to 1 quart of warm water); most commercial mouth washes should be avoided as they contain alcohol.

- Radiation to the jaws will also affect the salivary glands so that they produce less saliva. If you develop a sore mouth, drink plenty of fluids and rinse your mouth out frequently to get rid of food debris which would normally be swallowed with saliva. Some patients find it useful to suck ice cubes. If the problem is chronic, fluoride mouth washes or artificial saliva can be used.

- A change in taste is common during radiotherapy to the mouth. This may be a simple loss of taste or may make certain foods unpleasant. Experiment with foods to see which taste best and try to prepare foods that look or smell good even if you cannot taste them.
- If the radiotherapy includes the scalp *temporary* hair loss occurs. This is very upsetting, and is difficult to adjust to, but the hair will start to grow back after treatment. Many patients have wigs whilst they have lost their hair (they are supplied by the National Health Service in Britain) and others wear hats or scarves.
- Radiation to the testes or ovaries will usually result in loss of fertility. The testes are specially sensitive to radiotherapy.

Other side-effects of radiotherapy are less common and depend on the area being treated and it is important to discuss possible side-effects with your radiotherapist before treatment.

Many patients understandably feel 'down' or depressed during treatment; this is probably a result of several factors. Worry about the diagnosis of cancer, and about the type of treatment, together with a sudden change in daily routine and the side-effects of the treatment, all cause depression. This is normal, but it is useful if you can discuss your feelings with relatives and friends as well as the doctors and nurses.

With all radiation there is a *small* long-term risk that the treatment itself may cause a second cancer. Such tumours are uncommon and usually do not occur for a number of years (up to 20 years).

QUESTIONS TO ASK ABOUT THE SIDE-EFFECTS OF RADIOTHERAPY

(1) Will I feel tired?
(2) Will I feel sick?

(3) Are there any specific side-effects caused by the particular type of radiotherapy I am receiving?

(4) How long will the side-effects last?

(5) Are any special precautions required?

(6) Are there any long-term effects of the treatment?

(7) Will the radiotherapy affect my fertility?

RADIATION IMPLANT THERAPY

When certain tumours are being treated a small container of radioactive material may be placed (implanted) into a patient's body. The way that the radioactive material is implanted depends on the area to be treated, and if you are to receive such a treatment it is important that you discuss it with your radiotherapist.

Patients are usually admitted to hospital for the procedure and an anaesthetic may be necessary. The stay in hospital varies but is often less than one week. Patients are usually in a single room to protect others from the radiation of the implant, and visiting is sometimes restricted and you may be asked to stay in bed so as not to displace the implant.

Side-effects depend on where the implant is and patients should ask their doctor about this. The radioactive implant will be removed before the patient goes home and is then no longer a risk to other people.

GENERAL QUESTIONS ABOUT RADIOTHERAPY

Discuss your treatment fully with your doctor before starting. It is sometimes useful to write the questions down before seeing a doctor and to make a note of answers.

(1) Why do I need radiotherapy?

(2) Are there alternative treatments?

(3) Which part of me will be treated with the radiation?

(4) How long will the treatment take?

(5) How often will the treatment be given?

(6) How long does each treatment take?

(7) Can I drive, or do I need transport home?

(8) What are the general or particular side-effects?

(9) Should I take any special precautions during treatment?

Patients having any difficulties during treatment should tell their doctor.

CHAPTER 12

Drug treatment
(chemotherapy) of cancer

Chemotherapy (a shortened name for chemical therapy) is the use of drugs and hormones to treat disease. Although the word can be applied to other drug treatments, it is commonly used to mean the drug treatment of cancer.

Only thirty years ago there were no useful drugs for the treatment of cancer. The speciality of chemotherapy or medical oncology (the medical or drug treatment of tumours) is therefore very new. From the first discovery of anticancer drugs in the late 1940s there has been a rapid development of drug therapy, and this continues.

The major drawback of surgery and radiotherapy is that they only treat locally. Chemotherapy treats the whole body and cancer which has spread is affected. Drug treatment is, however, often given in combination with surgery of radiotherapy.

HOW DO THE DRUGS WORK?

It is beyond the scope of this book to describe in detail the way each type of drug works. There are more than thirty commonly used anticancer drugs, and each works in a different way though they often fall into broad groups or classes acting similarly. A list of the common classes of drugs, their uses and common side-effects are shown in Appendix A (page 303).

- In general, cancer drugs work by poisoning cells. They damage or kill cells, so that they are unable to divide and multiply, and unfortunately they harm both normal and cancer cells. Despite major efforts, we have failed to develop drugs which only attack cancerous cells and successful treatment depends on damaging tumour cells more than normal cells.

- High doses damage more cells. Medical oncologists frequently use high doses of drugs to kill as many tumour cells as possible; this will, of course, cause side-effects. If high-dose treatment can cure or greatly prolong life then most doctors and patients feel that it is worthwhile; but for tumours that do not respond well to chemotherapy, toxic treatment should be avoided as it may do more harm than good.

- Most anticancer drugs kill or damage cells best when the cells are dividing. The normal cells in the body that divide rapidly are in the bone marrow (making new blood), in the bowel (making new lining cells), in the hair follicles, in the testis (making sperm), and in the skin. Because of this, the common side-effects (page 86) of chemotherapy mainly affect these parts of the body. Many cancers have cells that are dividing rapidly, though this alone does not explain the effectiveness of anticancer drugs and, unfortunately, there are also cells within tumours that are not dividing. Some drugs will attack these cells and scientists are looking for more drugs that will do this.

- The larger a cancer is the slower its cells are dividing. Since drugs are most effective against rapidly dividing cells it is only to be expected that anticancer drugs are most useful in small tumours. Because the blood supply of large tumours is poor, the ability of drugs to get into a big tumour is also affected. These two factors mean that chemotherapy is best given when tumours have not grown to a large size though it does not mean that drugs cannot be effective in a large responsive tumour, only that the chances are reduced.

- During the early years of chemotherapy single drugs were commonly used alone. Despite some effect, tumours usually grew back and drugs are now usually used together in a combination. It is thought that single drugs fail because the cancer develops a way of overcoming their effects. This is less likely if several drugs, working in different ways, are used together. As well as choosing drugs that act differently, doctors try to put together drugs that have different side-effects so that high doses of all the drugs can be given.

- So that big doses of the drugs can be used treatment is only given once every few weeks. Some treatments, especially those taken by mouth, may be given continuously.

WHEN SHOULD CHEMOTHERAPY BE USED?

The drugs used in cancer chemotherapy probably cause more side-effects than any other medicines. For this reason it is very important that they are only used when they will benefit the patient.

If the treatment is likely to be curative, then chemotherapy that causes side-effects is usually acceptable both to the patient and doctor. It is more difficult to decide if chemotherapy is helpful when the chance of a good response is small or if the aim of the treatment is purely to relieve symptoms (palliative treatment). When doctors and patients consider drug treatment of cancer they must always weigh the potential advantages of the treatment against the side-effects. Such a balance is frequently complex, and you should discuss the need for treatment, its aims and disadvantages. The effectiveness of chemotherapy is changing rapidly and patients *must* discuss their own particular treatment with their doctor.

Cancers that can be cured with chemotherapy

There is a small but growing list of cancers that can be cured with drugs used alone or together with other treatments. These include acute lymphatic leukaemia in children. Wilm's tumour in children (a kidney cancer), rhabdomyosarcoma in children (a tumour of muscle), osteogenic sarcoma in children (a tumour of bones), lymphomas in children (cancer of lymph glands), Hodgkin's disease (a cancer of lymph glands), testicular cancer, chorio-carcinoma in women (cancer of the tissue of the placenta after child birth), lymphomas in adults (cancer of the lymph glands).

Most of the cancers on this list are relatively uncommon. The treatment of several includes hospital admission and a lot of drug side-effects but most patients will accept these disadvantages for a chance of cure.

Chemotherapy that reduces symptoms or prolongs life (palliation)

Many advanced tumours cannot, yet, be cured by chemo-therapy. Relief of symptoms and prolongation of life is,

however, possible in some of these cancers. If palliative chemotherapy is planned then there must be a clear goal; the trade-
off in terms of toxic side-effects must be worthwhile. Toxicity
is discussed more fully later in this chapter, but if palliative
treatment is to be given a thorough discussion of side-effects is
essential. Chemotherapy may be of some benefit in the following cancers: almost all childhood cancers if not curable will
respond to drugs; cancer of the breast; cancer of the ovary; oat
cell (small cell) cancer of the lung; acute leukaemia in adults;
multiple myeloma; cancer of the prostate; cancer of the thyroid;
some adult sarcomas; and cancer of the pancreas.

Cancers that do not respond to chemotherapy

Chemotherapy is not very effective in some of the common
cancers. This is not to say that they never respond; only that
useful antitumour effects are infrequent. When the benefits of
chemotherapy are uncertain the side-effects of treatment must
be considered with great care. If there is no curative treatment,
then only therapy which has few side-effects should be
considered, unless patients are willing or anxious to be treated
with new experimental drugs.

The following cancers often respond poorly to chemotherapy:
cancers of the colon and rectum, oesophagus, stomach, mouth,
bladder, cervix and brain; non-small cell lung cancer (page 171);
and malignant melanoma. Occasionally patients do benefit from
treatment; those most likely to respond are patients who feel
well before treatment and who have relatively small tumours.
Large tumours in very sick patients almost never respond usefully to chemotherapy and drug treatment is best avoided in
such patients. The tumours on these lists are gradually changing
and with time more tumours will become treatable and eventually curable.

HOW IS CHEMOTHERAPY GIVEN?

Anticancer chemotherapy is usually given in one of three ways.
(a) By mouth, some drugs are given as tablets or capsules.
(b) Intramuscularly, a *few* drugs are given by injection into a
    muscle or under the skin.
(c) Intravenously, many of the drugs are given by an injection

into a vein on the forearm. A small needle is put through the skin into a vein and the drug solution injected slowly (Figure 25). This should be relatively painless though it can become difficult to find 'easy' veins in patients who have had a lot of chemotherapy.

- When some drugs are given the needle in the vein is connected to a bottle containing a salt solution (an infusion) and the drug is then injected into the fluid running into the vein. Occasionally the drug may be mixed with the solution in the bottle and allowed to run slowly into the vein over a longer period.

- Many patients ask if chemotherapy is painful. On the whole the answer is no. Occasionally, the intravenous injection of certain drugs may cause a burning sensation in the vein and a mild pain may last for some hours after treatment. Putting the intravenous needle into a vein should be quite easy in most patients, but as treatment progresses the veins may be damaged by repeated injections so that it becomes more difficult to get a needle in the vein. Tell your doctor or nurse of any pain experienced when a drug is being injected. This may be a sign to stop the injection as some drugs damage the skin if they leak from the vein.

- If you are to have a long and complicated course of drugs, or if treatment becomes difficult to give, a long plastic line or catheter may be placed in a larger vein. Recently special catheters have made treatment easier for some patients. The major advantage of these catheters is that they can be left in place throughout the treatment. All drugs, transfusions, etc. can be given through this line and blood can be withdrawn for tests. Disadvantages include the small operation required to put it in and the scrupulous care required to prevent infection or clotting in the catheter. Nevertheless, it may be of benefit to patients receiving intensive treatment or those who have very poor veins in their arms. Not all centres use these lines, but they are becoming more commonly used when a patient is about to start a period of intensive treatment.

- Slow infusions of drugs are given to some patients and small portable pumps are becoming available. A needle is placed in a vein as usual and is connected by a short

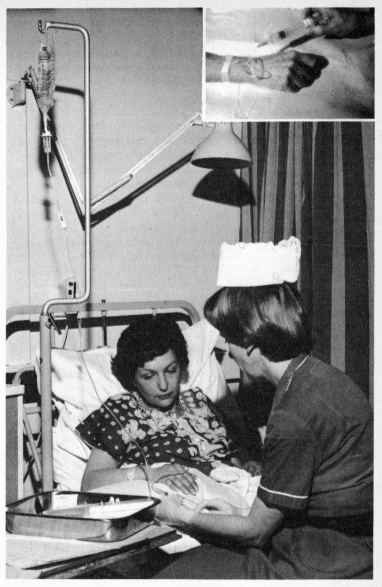

Figure 25 A patient being given a chemotherapy drug into a vein. An intra-venous infusion (drip) is set up and the drug is injected into the fluid running into a vein on the arm. The inset photograph shows a small needle, known as a butterfly, being used for an injection into a vein on the forearm

plastic line to a pump containing the drug; this injects the drug slowly at the required rate. This is a recent development that is being used more commonly.

WHAT ARE THE SIDE-EFFECTS OF CHEMOTHERAPY?

Side-effects vary from drug to drug and person to person. Not everyone will have side-effects and it is important that a doctor or nurse explains the sort of toxicity that you can expect. This may be minimal or quite severe, depending on the drugs given. However, even when patients are told that the side-effects may be severe, some may be lucky and get away with little inconvenience. The more common side-effects are discussed in this section; remember this is a list, you must discuss the *specific* effects of the therapy you will receive. Appendix A includes the common side-effects of the major anticancer drugs. It is also important to ask if you will be able to work or carry on as normal during treatment. Experience will allow the doctor to give a fairly accurate assessment of what to expect, but patients have a better idea after the first treatment as the pattern of side-effects is usually similar with each course.

Tiredness and malaise

Many patients feel tired and unwell, 'one degree under' is a common description. This may gradually get worse during the treatment, though it commonly improves between each course or cycle of treatment.

Decreased appetite, nausea and vomiting

One of the most troublesome side-effects cause by some anticancer drugs is nausea and vomiting. Patients will be given treatment (tablets, suppositories, or possibly injections) to help control the nausea. If you develop this side-effect, it usually starts within a few hours of treatment and is over by 12 hours; occasional patients may be nauseated for several days. The drugs which most frequently cause nausea and vomiting (see Appendix A) are cisplatin, nitrogen mustard, adriamycin, cyclophosphamide, CCNU, BCNU, actinomycin D; daunomycin, and DTIC. The severity of the nausea varies markedly between patients but if vomiting is very severe patients may need to be hospitalized to prevent dehydration and to make sure that the best antisickness treatment is given.

Patients may be able to help minimize the sickness at home by observing the following points:

(1) Eat small frequent meals for a day or so after treatment.
(2) Don't drink liquids with meals, so as not to overfill the stomach. Drink frequent small amounts of clear fluids between meals.
(3) Avoid spicy, fried, or fatty foods.
(4) Eat slowly and chew the food well so that it is easily digested.
(5) Only eat a light meal before chemotherapy.

If nausea and vomiting is a problem, tell your chemotherapy nurse and doctor. Alternative antisickness treatment may be helpful.

Sore mouth (mucositis or stomatitis)

Some drugs damage the cells lining the mouth and cause soreness and ulceration. As you may be prone to develop infections, it is very important to take care of your mouth if it becomes sore.

Good mouth care includes: (1) Regular brushing of teeth (up to 4 times per day) with a soft, round bristle toothbrush. (2) Mouth washes after each brushing. A mixture of 1 teaspoon of baking soda to one cup of warm water may be used. Commercial mouth washes containing alcohol should be avoided. (3) The use of dental floss between the teeth as well as brushing. (4) If soreness becomes severe or white patches develop in your mouth, see your doctor as you may have thrush (an infection with a fungus called candida). This requires intensive treatment with antifungal mouth washes or lozenges as well as the usual mouth care. (5) Avoid alcohol and spicy foods (including salt) that may cause a burning sensation. (6) Eat soft foods; try putting normal foods in a blender, and make sure there is plenty of gravy to moisten them.

The drugs that most commonly cause mucositis (Appendix A) are methotrexate, bleomycin, adriamycin, and daunomycin.

Diarrhoea

Diarrhoea is sometimes a problem. Doctors should be able to give medicines for this but you can help it by the following means. (1) Eat warm foods rather than hot (hot food speeds up the bowel movements). (2) Avoid foods high in fibre; these include raw fruits and vegetables, whole grain cereals and nuts. (3) Avoid gassy foods such as cabbage, cauliflower, and baked beans. The drugs that most commonly cause diarrhoea are 5-fluorouracil and cisplatin (Appendix A).

Bone marrow suppression or low blood counts

The bone marrow is the site where the body makes the cells that circulate in the blood. Red blood cells prevent anaemia and carry oxygen around the body. White blood cells fight infections and the platelets help the blood to clot. Because the bone marrow cells that make these three types of blood cells are dividing rapidly (page 81) they are frequently damaged by chemotherapy. This damage is temporary, but it is common for the cells in the blood (measured by a blood count) to drop to low levels for a week or so after each treatment and doctors will ask for a blood count before each treatment to ensure that your blood count is at a safe level to continue treatment. If the level of the white cells or platelets is too low, chemotherapy may be delayed a week or the dose of drugs reduced. If you become anaemic (too few red cells) a blood transfusion will be given.

- The degree to which the blood counts drops depends very much on the intensity and type of treatment. If you have a low white count, take precautions to help prevent an infection. (1) Avoid crowds or people with contagious diseases (those caught through close contact). (2) Take great care in cutting your nails and caring for the cuticles. (3) Wear protective gloves if gardening or doing any dirty jobs. Despite this you can still develop an infection as some of the normal bacteria (germs) living in the body may become agressive and attack the body when its normal defence mechanisms are damaged. If you develop the following symptoms, see your doctor *quickly*: (a) temperature (fever) over 100° Fahrenheit, (b) feeling hot or cold and shivering (rigors), (c) frequency and burning on passing urine, (d) cough, (e) diarrhoea for more than 2 days.

If you do develop an infection whilst your blood count is low, see a doctor immediately; as urgent and intensive antibiotic treatment in hospital may be necessary. It is dangerous to ignore an infection when your blood count is low.

- Platelets (the clotting cells in the blood) can fall to low levels after treatment so that you may bruise or bleed even with the slightest injury. If you have abnormal bleeding (nose bleeds, bleeding gums, blood in urine or faeces), or easy bruising or tiny red spots under the skin (bleeding spots called petechiae) contact your doctor immediately.

  A transfusion of platelets may be needed. These can be repeated until the platelets return to normal. Patients whose platelets are low should observe the following points.

  (1) Avoid injury, and if you do cut yourself apply firm pressure with a clean cloth for several minutes. If this does not stop the bleeding call your doctor.

  (2) Do not garden.

  (3) Do not use any aspirin-containing drugs (check *all* drugs labels for aspirin), as aspirin damages platelets.

  (4) Do not drink alcohol.

- Patients with a low red cell count are anaemic and may develop the following symptoms: (1) tiredness and irritability, (2) dizziness, especially on exertion or when standing up suddenly, (3) shortness of breath, (4) feeling cold. If you develop these symptoms tell your doctor: a blood transfusion will make you feel much better if you are anaemic.

Hair loss

Cells in the hair follicles divide rapidly and may be affected by some types of chemotherapy. As a result scalp and body hair are commonly lost *temporarily* during treatment. Loss of hair is called alopecia. Losing your hair is very upsetting though most patients make a brave adjustment; some people like to cover their head whilst others prefer not to. Wigs are available on the National Health Service in Britain (it is advisable to order a wig at the start of treatment so that it can be matched to your own hair) though some patients use a scarf or cap. Hair usually begins to fall out about 2–3 weeks after the first treatment and with two drugs (adriamycin and daunorubicin) the loss is complete, though it is variable with other drugs. When hair comes out quickly it can be messy, so some patients wear a hair net in bed to stop it getting everywhere. The hair may start to grow back slightly during treatment and will gradually regrow after treatment has stopped. Often the new hair is thicker, curlier and sometimes darker or greyer than before. Although loss of scalp hair is most obvious, other body hair including pubic hair is frequently lost. The drugs (Appendix A) that most commonly cause hair loss are: adriamycin and daunorubicin (nearly *always* causing temporary complete hair loss), cyclophosphamide, 5-FU, actinomycin D; vincristine, and etoposide. Attempts to reduce hair loss with scalp torniquets (a tight band round the head to reduce scalp blood flow) and by freezing the scalp have been partially successful. It must be remembered that not all drugs cause hair loss and patients in doubt should ask their doctor.

Skin effects

Allergic skin rashes may develop during treatment. These are usually red, raised itchy rashes which are often over much of the body. Doctors can give tablets to reduce the symptoms and will try to find out which drug caused the rash. Any drug can cause a rash but procarbazine (Appendix A) is the chemotherapy drug which most commonly causes allergic rashes.

Anticancer drugs may also irritate veins around the place where they were injected. This may be uncomfortable and there may be a red or dark line over the vein. Bleomycin (Appendix A) often causes increased skin pigmentation (tanning) which is most intense at pressure points so that the elbows are often pigmented, as are any scratch marks. Busulphan (Appendix A) can also cause some skin pigmentation.

Nail changes may occur with many drugs. Because of slowing of nail growth during each treatment there may be white lines in the nails corresponding with each treatment. Nails may also flake or break easily.

Some drugs may damage the skin and underlying tissues if allowed to leak from the vein when they are being injected. If this happens it usually causes pain, and if you feel any pain during an injection into a vein, tell the nurse or doctor immediately so that the injection can be stopped. Even small amounts of drug that have leaked can cause a sore or ulcer which is very difficult to heal. The drugs (Appendix A) that can cause this side-effect are adriamycin, daunorubicin, actinomycin D, vincristine, vinblastine, and nitrogen mustard.

Nerves and muscles

Three drugs (vinblastine, vincristine and vindesine — Appendix A) frequently affect nerves relaying sensation to the brain and nerves controlling muscles. The commonest side-effect is pins and needles (called paraesthesia) affecting the fingers and toes. Nearly all patients receiving these drugs will notice some effects. If the symptoms progress to affect the whole hand or foot or cause difficulty in holding small objects, tell your doctor. Weakness in the hands and legs can be caused by these drugs and it is important that the chemotherapy nurse or doctor knows of any muscle weakness as the dose of the drug will need to be reduced or the drug stopped. 'Pins and needles' and minor muscle weakness usually clear up gradually over the first few months after treatment has stopped. Occasionally other drugs (especially cisplatin) can cause similar symptoms.

Muscle weakness, by itself, is common after high doses of steroids (Appendix A); the weakness recovers when the drug is stopped but in a few patients may be marked.

Ovarian and testicular effects

Women having menstrual periods often develop irregular periods and may stop having periods altogether (amenorrhoea) during chemotherapy. Menopausal symptoms (hot flushes, etc.) may result from treatment. When chemotherapy is stopped menstruation often returns to normal and periods follow their previous pattern. Occasionally, when menstrual periods have stopped altogether during chemotherapy they may fail to return to normal. This usually happens in women over 30 years of age and the drugs bring menopause on early. Despite abnormal periods during chemotherapy you could still become pregnant and should use birth control methods. The 'pill' is not recommended and if is worth discussing contraception with your doctor. Anticancer drugs can damage an unborn baby and care to avoid pregnancy is *important*.

The eggs (ova) in the ovary are formed before birth and one matures with each menstrual cycle. The eggs are not damaged by chemotherapy so that fertility may return to normal (provided that periods return) after the chemotherapy has stopped. Many women who have been treated with chemotherapy have subsequently become pregnant. The number of patients whose periods do not return normally has not been carefully studied for each type of drug treatment, so you should discuss the possible effects of your treatment on fertility. Reduced fertility is more common if chemotherapy has been given together with radiotherapy to the lower abdomen.

Chemotherapy in men is much more likely to damage the ability of the testis to make new sperm. Unlike the ovaries the testes are constantly making sperm and because the cells are dividing rapidly they are very susceptible to anticancer drugs. Not all drugs damage the testes (the alkylating agents (Appendix A) are the main culprits), and some men remain fertile despite intensive chemotherapy. If the testes are severely damaged it is likely to be a permanent effect and the incidence of sterility is very high with certain drug combinations, so it is important to discuss this with your doctor. Some hospitals have the facilities for storing sperm at very low temperatures (in liquid nitrogen), which allows the option of subsequent artificial insemination.

Although some patients may become sterile the chemotherapy should not interfere with your sex life. Hormones produced by the testes are not affected by chemotherapy, though stress and tiredness and general malaise of the treatment may temporarily lessen desire (libido) for sex.

Chemotherapy in pregnancy

Chemotherapy can damage an unborn baby (foetus). The risk is greatest during the first three months and doctors usually advise a therapeutic abortion for women treated with anticancer drugs during the first part of a pregnancy. Although chemotherapy may be damaging later in pregnancy, and these drugs are best avoided throughout pregnancy, normal babies have been born to women who received chemotherapy late in pregnancy. If you have *any* reason to think that you may be pregnant before or during treatment tell your doctor so that a pregnancy test can be arranged.

Effects on urine

Some drugs, notably adriamycin, daunorubicin (red) and mito-zantrone (blue), colour the urine for a few hours after treatment. Cyclophosphamide and a new related drug (Ifosphamide) may cause a chemical cystitis (inflammation of the bladder). The drug is broken down by the body into compounds which irritate the bladder when there are large amounts in the urine. If you receive these drugs you should increase your fluid intake (to at least 4 pints per day) for a day or two after treatment. Ifos-phamide is usually given with drug called Mesna in order to prevent cystitis. The symptoms of cystitis are discomfort or burning on passing urine, increased frequency of passing urine and blood in the urine. If you have these symptoms, contact your doctor immediately. The symptoms usually stop when drug treatment is discontinued but may become troublesome if it is continued or repeated.

Chemotherapy and other drugs

Some drugs may affect treatment (interact) with anticancer drugs. If you are taking any of the following drugs, tell your doctor.

    Antibiotics
    Anticoagulants (drugs to thin the blood and prevent clots)
    Anticonvulsants (drugs to prevent seizures in epilepsy)
    Aspirin (check all patent medicines which may contain aspirin)
    Barbiturates (rarely used sleeping pills)
    Blood pressure tablets
    Diabetic drugs
    Dieuretics (water tablets)
    Hormone pills (including contraceptive pills)
    Nasal sprays (decongestants)
    Sleeping pills
    Tranquillizers (Valium, etc.)
    Immunizations or vaccines. Live vaccines (e.g. yellow fever jab) should **never** be given to patients receiving anticancer

drugs. Always tell your doctor that you are on chemo-therapy before an immunization.

Increased risk of cancer

Many of the anticancer drugs are carcinogens (page 2), chemicals which can cause cancer, and patients treated with and cured by chemotherapy have a slightly increased risk of a second cancer. This risk is, however, small compared with the benefit of curative chemotherapy, and is highest in patients receiving both chemotherapy and radiotherapy.

Other side-effects

Most of the side-effects already discussed are general and you should ask about any particular side-effects caused by individual drugs (see common side-effects of the drugs in Appendix A).

WHEN SHOULD YOU CALL YOUR DOCTOR ABOUT SIDE-EFFECTS?

It is important to contact a doctor *early* if you have *any* worrying side-effects. Some complications can become serious if not tre-ated promptly and correctly; others are much less important and you can be reassured. Early contact with a doctor will reduce worry about symptoms and will identify the side-effects which require more urgent treatment.

EMOTIONAL EFFECTS

Undergoing cancer therapy is very stressful and highly emotional for most patients. Family and friends should under-stand that feelings like anger, depression, fear and apathy are to be expected (see Chapter 51 on communication). In addition to the stresses of the treatment itself, some drugs (particularly high dose steroids) can occasionally cause emotional upsets by themselves. Supportive therapy during this period is important and in addition to family and friends it is useful if you can talk over your problems and fears with your doctors and nurses. If you have found the diagnosis and treatment especially emotion-ally traumatic, it can be helpful to talk to a psychiatrist or psychotherapist or someone else skilled in this sort of problem. There really should be no stigma attached to these emotional problems; all patients have them to some degree. One of the most depressing features of treatment given in monthly cycles is that, just as you are getting back to normal, the next treatment, with its attendant side-effects, comes around.

QUESTIONS TO ASK ABOUT CHEMOTHERAPY

(1) Why is drug treatment necessary?
(2) What are the aims of chemotherapy?
(3) How are the drugs given?
(4) Are there any immediate side-effects?
(5) Do I need to go into hospital for treatment?
(6) If not, can I drive home afterwards?
(7) How often is the treatment given?
(8) How long does each treatment take?
(9) How many courses of treatment are planned? (If given, as tablets, continuously, what is the duration of treatment?)
(10) Are there any later side-effects (in particular does it affect fertility)?
(11) Should I take any special precautions before or after chemotherapy?
(12) How can I contact the hospital in case of worrying side-effects?

CHAPTER 13

Cancer of the stomach

Cancers of the stomach (Figure 26) have become less common in Western countries during the past forty years. It is a disease of late middle age (50–70 years) and is more common in heavy drinkers and sufferers from pernicious anaemia (lack of vitamin B_{12}); no other predisposing factors are known.

SYMPTOMS

The symptoms of stomach cancer are similar to those of an ulcer and include:

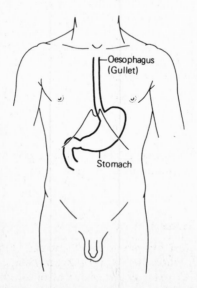

Figure 26 Diagrammatic representation of the upper gastrointestinal tract showing the position of the stomach

- Indigestion or upper abdominal pains; these may be helped by antacids, by eating, or by drinking milk.
- Vomit containing blood.
- Loss of appetite or weight.

Unfortunately many stomach cancers do not produce symptoms till they are quite far advanced. Any indigestion that does not clear quickly should be taken seriously and the advice of a doctor sought.

DIAGNOSIS

If you have persistent upper abdominal pains or any of the above symptoms, you should have investigations to find out the cause. In most cases cancer is not found, but it is important to be sure.

The tests used include:

- A barium meal (page 30). In this test a white liquid is swallowed; this shows up on an X-ray, outlining the stomach.
- Gastroscopy (page 61). In this test a special flexible instrument is swallowed and is used to look into the stomach. If a suspicious area is seen, a small piece (a biopsy) can be taken for examination under a microscope.
- Other tests may include a chest X-ray, blood tests and, if a cancer is found, a liver scan (page 50) or possibly a CT body scan (page 47).

TREATMENT

Unfortunately, stomach cancer is frequently not diagnosed till it has become quite advanced and many patients die of the tumour.

Surgery (Chapter 10)

This is the most important treatment and may be curative in some patients whose disease is at an early stage. Operations for stomach cancer may require removal of all or a large part of the stomach and its local lymph glands (page 23). Patients who have had such an operation (radical or total gastrectomy) usually need a special diet consisting of regular small amounts of foods that are high in protein and fat but low in sugar. Regular injections of vitamin B_{12} may also be required. It is usually necessary to make a vertical incision (cut) over the upper abdomen and following the operation tubes or drains may be left temporarily in the abdomen to remove any blood or fluid. Patients will be up soon after the operation and should be able to leave hospital after 10–14 days.

Unfortunately in many patients the tumour is too advanced for such an operation to be helpful.

Radiotherapy (Chapter 11)

This is not routinely used for the treatment of stomach cancer though it may be helpful in dealing with symptoms, such as pain, caused by secondary spread.

Chemotherapy (Chapter 12)

Although some drugs are helpful in stomach cancer they cannot cure advanced disease. The drug most commonly used is 5-FU, alone or in combination with adriamycin or mitomycin C (Appendix A). About a quarter of patients treated with chemotherapy have a useful response but only a few patients respond for a long time. In cases of advanced stomach cancer there are three possible approaches to the tumour: (1) no anti-cancer treatment, apart from therapy for specific symptoms, (2) a simple treatment with few side-effects (such as 5-FU), and (3) patients may be included in a trial of combination chemotherapy. There are no clear rules for the treatment of advanced stomach cancer but it is probably best to avoid drug combinations in patients who are very unwell from their tumour. Combination chemotherapy remains unproven and ideally should be used only in trials testing its usefulness. In patients with a small tumour, combination chemotherapy (adjuvant therapy, page 125) after surgery is being tested, but the results do not yet support the routine use of such treatment.

SUMMARY OF TREATMENT OF STOMACH CANCER

(1) Stomach cancer is becoming less common in Western countries and screening is not helpful.
(2) Unexplained indigestion or ulcer symptoms should be investigated.
(3) Surgery is potentially curative but most patients already have extensive disease that cannot be treated by surgery.
(4) Radiotherapy may be used to control symptoms.
(5) Drug therapy may consist of 5-FU alone or in combination with adriamycin and mitomycin C, but is only useful in about a quarter of patients.
(6) Adjuvant chemotherapy is not of proven value and trials continue.

CHAPTER 14

Cancer of the pancreas

The pancreas is a gland that lies below the stomach and along-side the first part of the bowel (Figure 27). It produces digestive enzymes and insulin. The digestive enzymes get into the bowel by a small tube called the pancreatic duct.

The pancreas lies deep in the abdomen and tumours of this gland are rarely diagnosed at an early stage when they are curable.

SYMPTOMS

There are no early symptoms and patients rarely notice anything wrong until the tumour is advanced and has invaded nearby organs. The main symptoms are:

• Pain in the upper abdomen and frequently in the back.

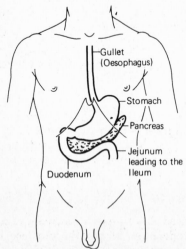

Figure 27 Diagrammatic representation of the upper gastrointestinal tract show-ing the position of the pancreas

- Weight loss.
- Loss of appetite.
- Jaundice (the accumulation of yellow bile pigment in the body which causes a yellow appearance of the whites of the eyes and the skin).

DIAGNOSIS

As the pancreas is such a deep-seated organ it is often difficult to make the diagnosis of pancreatic cancer. The usual tests include:

- Barium meal (page 30) to see if the pancreas is enlarged and is pressing on the duodenum (see Figure 27).
- Ultrasound examination (page 45) of the upper abdomen to see if there is a lump in the region of the pancreas.
- CT body scan (page 47), will also show if there is a lump in this area.
- Endoscopy (page 63). including ERCP, allows the doctor to examine the pancreatic duct as it enters the bowel and to pass a fine tube into the duct so that some contrast dye can be injected and an X-ray picture taken.
- Very occasionally an arteriogram (page 41) may be done to outline the blood vessels in the gland.

As it may be difficult to be certain of the diagnosis of pancreatic cancer it is often necessary to do several of these tests.

TREATMENT

Unfortunately, in most patients the tumour is too far advanced at diagnosis for there to be a hope of cure, but treatment to control the tumour or relieve symptoms can be given.

Surgery (Chapter 10)

If the tests discussed above suggest pancreatic cancer an exploratory abdominal operation (a laparotomy) is usually performed. A biopsy is taken to prove the diagnosis if cancer is suspected; a careful assessment for any possible spread in the abdomen is then made. In most patients tumour is found beyond the pancreas and surgery is palliative (page 68), being designed to prevent further symptoms. The main aim is to prevent obstruction of the bile duct (this would cause jaundice)or of the bowel. Occasionally the tumour appears to be confined to the pancreatic gland and a surgical operation to remove the pancreas may be planned. This operation (a Whipples procedure or radical pancreatectomy) is technically difficult, even when done by an experienced surgeon.

Some surgeons doubt that a Whipples procedure is ever very helpful, but it may be useful when done on very carefully selected patinets who have small tumours and who are in good general health. After a Whipples procedure patients will, like diabetics, require insulin replacement therapy.

Radiation therapy (Chapter 11)

Radiotherapy may be useful for treating some of the symptoms of pancreatic cancer, but cure is very unlikely. Trials of radiotherapy in the treatment of pancreatic cancer are being run at present.

Chemotherapy (Chapter 12)

Anticancer drug therapy is of limited value as only about a quarter of the patients respond and the responses are only temporary. 5-FU is the most frequently used drug but several other drugs may be used (including adriamycin and mitomycin C — Appendix A). Combination drug therapy should ideally only be used in trials as its role remains undefined. Although most patients do not benefit from chemotherapy, occasional good responses do occur.

It is important if a pancreatic cancer is found to discuss the aims of treatment at the outset. Cure is only occasionally possible and treatment is usually designed to prevent symptoms and prolong life.

SUMMARY OF THE TREATMENT OF PANCREATIC CANCER

(1) Pancreatic cancer is usually found at a late stage.

(2) It may be difficult to make the diagnosis.
(3) Surgery is usually palliative (designed to prevent symptoms).
(4) Occasionally radical removal of the pancreas may be curative.
(5) Radiotherapy is only useful for controlling symptoms.
(6) Chemotherapy is not very active in this tumour. Combination chemotherapy has shown early promise but is best used in trials.

CHAPTER 15

Liver cancer

There is often confusion between cancers that have developed elsewhere, the bowel for example, and subsequently spread to the liver and cancers developing in the liver itself. Spread to the liver (secondary cancer) is common whilst primary liver cancers are rare in Western counties. Only cancers *developing* in the liver should normally be called liver cancer and this section only deals with these tumours.

Some liver cancers may be caused by exposure to chemicals and vinyl chloride is known to have caused some tumours. Some male hormones (testosterone) and the oral contraceptive pill cause liver tumours, though many of these are benign and the risk is very small. Liver cancer is more common in people who have alcoholic cirrhosis and over half the cases of liver cancer in the West are associated with cirrhosis.

SYMPTOMS

These are often vague and include;

- Weakness.
- Loss of appetite.
- Abdominal discomfort or pain.
- Bloated abdomen.

The diagnosis may be complicated by an underlying cirrhosis which can cause similar symptoms itself.

DIAGNOSIS

A biopsy of the liver is usually necessary (page 00). The best area to biopsy may be shown by examining the liver with:

- Liver scan (page 55).
- Liver ultrasound (page 45).

TREATMENT

Unfortunately, the outlook is usually very poor. The only chance for cure depends on the rare finding of a cancer localized to one part of the liver. If this is the case then surgery to remove part of the liver, if the patient is fit enough, is attempted. This type of surgery should, preferably, only be done by a surgeon experienced in this field. Liver transplants are still experimental and are usually only possible if there is no sign of cancer outside the liver. Secondary tumours that have spread from elsewhere cannot be treated in this way.

Radiation or chemotherapy to help symptoms can be given to patients who cannot undergo surgery. Treatment is palliative and unfortunately many patients die within one year.

CHAPTER 16

Cancer of the oesophagus (gullet)

The oesophagus is the tube that connects the mouth to the stomach (Figure 28). Rhythmic contractions of muscles in the wall of the oesophagus pass food and liquid into the stomach when swallowing.

In the West the most important predisposing factor is heavy alcohol use. The tumour may also occur in patients with other chronic and long-term benign conditions affecting the oesophagus. These include: (1) The Plummer–Vinson syndrome which is a condition in young women where there is anaemia, difficulty in swallowing, and a web of tissue in the oesophagus. It is

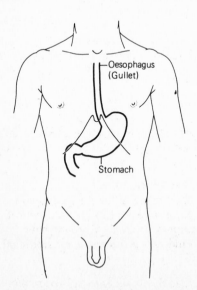

Figure 28 Diagrammatic representation of the upper gastrointestinal tract showing the course of the oesophagus (gullet)

usually improved or cured by an adequate diet and iron supplements. The syndrome may also be known as the Kelly–Patterson or Sideropenic syndrome. (2) Achalasia (loss of the normal rhythmic contractions of the gullet that aid swallowing) results in relaxation of the oesophageal walls and a ballooning of the oesophagus which contains fluid and undigested food particles. The resulting chronic inflammation predisposes to cancer. Operations can correct achalasia. (3) Cancer is also more common in patients who have a stricture of the gullet caused by swallowing caustic liquids.

Routine screening is not justified in Western countries.

SYMPTOMS

This is a tumour that usually causes symptoms late in its course. The commonest complaints include:

- Difficulty in swallowing. This is initially on eating solids and later on swallowing fluids. This difficulty is often intermittent but is progressive.
- Pain in the chest or back.
- Weight loss.
- Anaemia caused by oozing loss of blood from the tumour.
- If the obstruction is severe, vomiting, which is often blood-stained, may occur.

DIAGNOSIS

This is usually straightforward and is made by X-ray and direct visual examination using an endoscope (Chapter 9). The test used are:

- Barium swallow (page 30).
- Oesophagoscopy using a flexible gastroscope (page 61). If a tumour is seen, a biopsy (a small specimen of tissue) will be taken for examination under a microscope.
  In patients found to have a tumour, additional tests include:

- Chest X-ray.
- Liver scan (page 50) or ultrasound (page 45).
- Blood tests of liver function.

TREATMENT

Unfortunately the tumour is usually at an advanced stage when the diagnosis is made so that curative surgery is often not possible. In addition only a quarter of tumours are in the lower part of the oesophagus where it is easier to perform an operation.

Surgery (Chapter 10)

Surgical removal of cancer from the lower third of the oesophagus is still technically difficult and only rarely cures patients. When it can be performed it restores normal swallowing. If on examination the tumour is not too big or fixed then a surgeon can remove the tumour and bring the stomach up into the chest and reconnect it to the upper part of the oesophagus. This is a major operation performed by a thoracic (chest) surgeon.

For tumours of the upper and middle parts of the oesophagus surgery is even more difficult. Operations designed to remove the tumour and then to bring part of the large bowel into the chest to reconnect the two ends of the oesophagus are occasionally done. The risk of complications and likelihood of death during or shortly after the operation are appreciable, and this sort of operation should only be considered in carefully selected cases where cure is the aim. This operation requires an incision (cut) over the chest and abdomen and a long recovery period is usually required. When an operation on the chest is performed drains are left in the chest for a few days to remove air or fluid.

Radiation therapy (Chapter 11)

Radiotherapy can be a useful palliative therapy (treatment for symptoms) in oesophageal cancer. It is the usual treatment for cancers of the upper oesophagus but may also be used for advanced cancers of the lower oesophagus.

Radiotherapy is given for 4 or 5 days each week for a total of 4–6 weeks. The first visit to the department is spent planning the individual treatment for the patient. Side-effects include:

- Some nausea.
- Loss of appetite.
- Irritation and reddening of the skin over the area being treated.

- Soreness on swallowing.

Radiotherapy is sometimes used together with surgery.

Chemotherapy (Chapter 12)

Although the tumour may spread to the liver, lungs and bone there are, unfortunately, no useful drugs in oesophageal cancer and routine chemotherapy is not recommended though trials of experimental drug therapy continue.

PALLIATIVE TREATMENT

As patients with oesophageal cancer may not be able to swallow, special ways of overcoming this have been designed. If a tumour is very advanced a special plastic tube may be pushed through it to open up the oesophagus.

This is done at a minor operation and dramatically relieves symptoms, allows normal eating and in advanced cases is of great help.

SUMMARY OF TREATMENT OF OESOPHAGEAL CANCER

(1) Screening is of no value except possibly in those with conditions predisposing to the tumour.
(2) It is usually diagnosed when it is already advanced.
(3) Surgery is rarely curative but is helpful in selected cases.
(4) Operations on the lower third are technically easier.
(5) Chemotherapy is ineffective.
(6) The insertion of a plastic tube through the cancer may give very effective relief of symptoms.

CHAPTER 17

Large bowel (colon or rectum) cancer

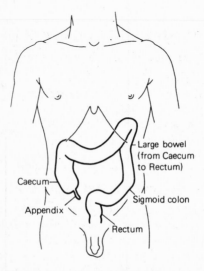

Figure 29 Diagrammatic representation of the course of the large bowel

Cancers of the large bowel or lower intestine are very probably associated with diet. In those countries where the people eat little fibre (roughage) but a lot of animal fats, protein, and refined sugar, the incidence is high, compared with that in places where plenty of fibre and little refined sugar or meat is eaten.

Diets low in fibre result in small stools and a slow transit time through the intestine. It has been suggested that the risk of cancer is higher if cancer-causing substances (carcinogens, page 2) in the stool are in contact with the bowel wall for a long time. This is more likely if transit is slow.

The way our Western diet may cause colon cancer is not proven, but a move towards a diet including more roughage and less animal fats and protein has been recommended by some doctors.

The colon is a muscular tube that starts at the right side of the abdomen; it is about 1.5 m long and ends at the anus. Descriptively it is divided into the several parts shown in Figure 29.

SYMPTOMS AND INVESTIGATIONS

The main symptoms of large bowel cancer are:

- Blood in the stools.
- Feeling of fullness or pain in the rectum.
- Difficulty in evacuating the bowel.
- Persistent constipation or diarrhoea.
- Thin stringy stools.
- Pain in the lower abdomen.
- Anaemia (due to lack of iron) without explanation.

Nearly all colon cancers bleed and investigation includes:

- Examination of the stool for blood.
- A rectal examination and general physical examination.
- Sigmoidoscopy (page 59) to look into the lower bowel and obtain a biopsy if possible.
- Barium enema (page 31) and possibly colonoscopy and biopsy (page 60).

If cancer is found, a chest X-ray, blood tests, and liver ultrasound (page 45) or isotope scan (page 50) should be done before surgery is planned. If these show spread of tumour it may alter surgical management.

TREATMENT

Surgery (Chapter 10)

Surgical removal of the tumour cures up to half of patients with colon cancer and is the most important treatment. During and after surgery the extent of tumour spread in the bowel is carefully looked at, as the likelihood of cure is closely related to the degree of spread or 'stage' of the cancer (Chapter 8). The staging system used for large bowel cancer is known as the 'Dukes classification'. If the cancer is confined to the lining (mucosa) of the bowel (Dukes' A) the chance of cure is very high. If the cancer has invaded into the muscle wall of the bowel (Dukes' B) the chances are intermediate whilst if the tumour has spread to local lymph nodes (Dukes' C) they are least good.

The type of operation used to remove the tumour varies from patient to patient. If the cancer is very close to the anus then it is impossible to remove the tumour and to join the ends of the bowel together, as incontinence will follow the operation. In such cases a colostomy (page 291) is performed. In this operation the rectum is removed and the colon is brought through the lower abdominal wall which is covered with a special bag to collect stool. It is, of course, always difficult to adjust to the idea of a colostomy, but most patients after initial worries manage well and lead a normal life. Special nurses (stoma nurses) trained in the care of colostomies help with the early adjustment and colostomy associations (see Appendix D) in Britain and the United States have volunteers (usually with colostomies themselves) who will help.

Most patients with bowel cancer do not require a colostomy as the bowel can be joined together when the tumour has been removed. Fewer patients have a colostomy these days as new techniques for joining the bowel together allow operations nearer to the lower end of the rectum. Occasionally patients only develop symptoms when a cancer of the bowel causes obstruction. In such cases a surgeon may initially perform a colostomy even though the tumour is not near the anus. After the effects of the obstruction have settled down (usually some months) the colostomy may be taken away and the ends of the bowel joined together again at a second operation.

Whether or not a colostomy is necessary, the very best chance of cure lies with surgery. The technique of the operation depends on where the tumour is and you should discuss which type of operation is being planned.

Radiation therapy (Chapter 11)

Recent trials have suggested that in patients at inreased risk of tumour recurrence (Dukes' stage B or C) radiation may reduce the frequency of relapse if the tumour arises in the last part of the colon (sigmoid colon) or rectum (Figure 29). The side-effects of radiotherapy include diarrhoea, loss of appetite, and tiredness. Treatment lasts about four weeks and is given 4 to 5 times each week, the first visit being used to plan the treatment for the individual patient. Radiotherapy has only been used in this way recently and may be given before or after an operation; it is not routinely used for tumours of the rest of the large bowel.

Chemotherapy (Chapter 12)

Drugs have been used to treated advanced bowel cancer for a number of years. One drug (5-fluorouracil — Appendix A) has been the mainstay of treatment and there is no evidence that adding other drugs to 5-FU improve on its activity. Unfortunately only about one in every five patients has a useful response to treatment, though 5-FU is relatively free of side-effects (Appendix A) and is well tolerated by most patients.

As the response to chemotherapy is not good it has not routinely been used as adjuvant therapy (page 125) after surgery. Trials of adjuvant treatment are taking place and there is some evidence that direct infusions of 5-FU into the liver may be useful.

In some patients with metastatic spread of cancer a course of 5-FU chemotherapy is warranted. If there is no response after several courses further treatment is not helpful. There are few good alternative drugs though some patients may be treated with new drugs in trials; unfortunately, none look promising at the moment.

SUMMARY

(1) People at *high risk* of colon cancer should probably have routine screening tests. Those at no obvious increased risk should seek medical advice if they develop any of the symptoms of large bowel cancer. Programmes of screening of normal populations continue but are unproven.
(2) Surgery is the mainstay of treatment and is curative in about half of patients. Patients having a colostomy should receive

help from stoma nurses and if necessary local colostomy groups.

(3) Radiation therapy with surgery may be helpful in cancers of the last part of the bowel. Treatment may be given before or after the surgery.

(4) Chemotherapy is not very helpful for advanced tumour. The most useful drug, 5-FU, is relatively free of side-effects and combinations of drugs are best avoided. Adjuvant chemotherapy is being tested. Preliminary evidence suggests that infusions of 5-FU directly into the liver may be helpful.

CHAPTER 18

Cancer of the breast

Breast cancer is the commonest cancer in women living in the Western world. Early diagnosis is important as a tumour confined to the breast can be cured. Screening for breast cancer (Chapter 5) remains unproven, though the evidence is becoming stronger in women over 50 years of age.

Women using self-examination (page 13) should be shown how to do it by someone experienced in the technique and if this cannot be arranged locally there are cancer organizations that can help (Appendix D). Self-examination should be done seven days after each period or in women after the menopause on the same day each month. Recommendations for mammography (a special breast X-ray) are discussed in the section on screening. The anatomy of the breast and the ways a cancer may spread to draining lymph nodes is shown in Figure 30.

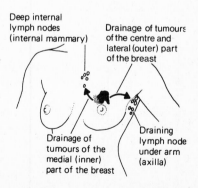

Figure 30 The routes of spread of breast cancer to lymph nodes

WHAT TO DO ABOUT A BREAST LUMP

Despite the apprehension that any women will feel on finding a breast lump, it is much better to see a doctor quickly. *MOST* lumps are not cancer at all and are harmless, but this can only be decided by an experienced doctor. Women who have had previous harmless lumps should not ignore a new lump—all lumps should be examined. General practitioners should refer all patients with a breast lump to a breast clinic or to those experienced in the care of breast disease and if your general practitioner takes no action about a lump ask for a second opinion; even experienced breast surgeons often cannot be sure a lump is benign without a biopsy. At the breast clinic, patients found to have a breast lump on examiantion, may have a mammogram (special X-ray of the breast—page 29) as the appearance of the lump can help the doctor to decide on further management. All patients, however, should have a biopsy if there is a persistent firm lump. Cystic (fluid-filled) lumps may be drained by sucking out the fluid with a syringe and needle. The fluid is then examined under 'a microscope to make sure that there are no malignant cells.

Some surgeons will do a breast biopsy under general anaesthetic and ask a pathologist to examine the tissue immediately (a frozen section) and if cancer is present will go on to perform a mastectomy (removal of the breast). Recently surgeons have begun to perform a biopsy, often under local anaesthetic, as a minor operation in a day ward. The biopsy tissue is examined by a pathologist after slower routine processing (this technique is more reliable than a frozen section) and if cancer is found a formal cancer operation is performed when the situation has been discussed with the patient. Such a biopsy may take the form of a small operation to remove the lump or the use of a special needle to remove a piece of the lump after a local anaesthetic has been given.

The major advantage of such an approach is that the need for, and surgical technique of, any cancer operation can be fully explained and agreed with the patient before it is done. There is no disadvantage in waiting for the result of a biopsy and many breast units now use this approach. If you wish to have this type of delayed operation ask for it. Many patients find it helpful to have a chance of adjusting to the new situation before undergoing an operation on their breast, and in those patients whose lump is not cancer (*the majority*) they will not have to suffer the agony of anticipating waking from the anaesthetic to find all or part of their breast gone.

TREATMENT

If the lump is malignant the care of breast cancer involves a team of doctors experienced in various branches of medicine and many centres have breast clinics that bring these doctors together. Although treatment has been standard in the past, there are now several areas of controversy. Patients should discuss the treatment options so that they know the advantages and disadvantages of each form of treatment. Although the main controversies are covered in this chapter, it is a complex field and you should take the opportunity to talk to your doctor about treatment.

Surgery (Chapter 10)

For a long time the usual operation for cancer of the breast was a Halstead radical mastectomy. This operation is disfiguring, as in addition to removal of the breast and lymph glands under

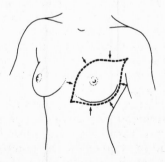

Figure 31 The type of incision (cut) used for the surgical removal of a breast (mastectomy)

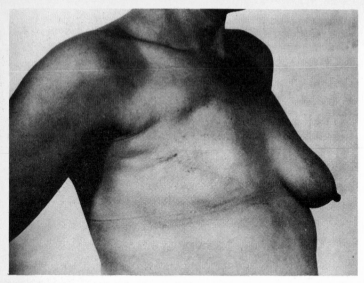

Figure 32 The scar left by the surgical removal of a breast (mastectomy)

the arm, a major part of the muscles on the front of the chest are removed. There is no evidence that this extensive operation is any better than operations not including removal of muscle.

Recently, a more acceptable alternative operation has been the modified radical or simple mastectomy. Whichever technique is used (there are minor technical differences) an incision (cut) is made and the breast and associated tissue (usually including the lymph nodes under the arm) are removed (Figure 31). The edges of the incision are stitched together so that a single scar remains (Figure 32). A suction drain is often left in the wound immediately after the operation to prevent fluid accumulating under the scar; these tubes are removed after a few days. Although the breast is sensitive, post-operative pain is not usually severe and is well controlled by pain medicines. Physiotherapy is given after the operation to ensure that the shoulder does not get stiff and patients should be out of bed the day after

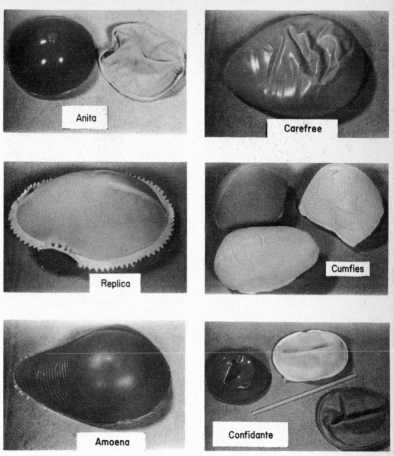

Figure 33 Different types of artificial breasts (prosthesis) currently used

the operation and the stitches are removed at 7–10 days, the patient is usually able to go home within one week.

Before leaving hospital patients should be given a light-weight breast prosthesis (artificial breast) to wear in the first few weeks after the operation. This restores the normal breast outline but does not exert pressure on the scar. Later you will be supplied

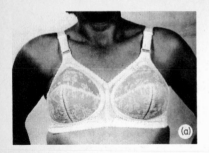 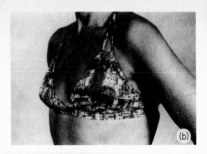

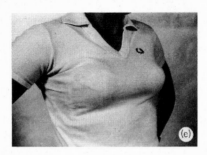

Figure 34 A woman who has had a mastectomy can wear various clothes with a prosthesis without it being visible: (a) bra, (b) bikini, (c) sports shirt

with a permanent breast prosthesis (Figure 33); some hospitals now have specialist mastectomy nurses who can help you with all your problems including choosing a prosthesis. A suitable comfortable bra is also important and despite understandable early anxiety many patients are able to wear low cut dresses and swim suits if they have a properly fitted prosthesis and choose their clothes sensibly (Figure 34).

Following a mastectomy there is inevitably a deep sense of

personal loss and many patients require time to adjust to the situation. The time required for adjustment varies considerably and is influenced not only by the patient's personality but also by the care and understanding she receives from the hospital and her family.

Women who have had a mastectomy can lead an active sex life. Sexual difficulties can occur but should not always be blamed purely on the mastectomy—such difficulties are not uncommon at times of stress and anxiety. Support at times of emotional difficulty can be provided by mastectomy nurses, breast clinics and groups such as the Mastectomy Association (page 315). Because women often do not complain of anxiety and depression to their doctor, mastectomy nurses or other trained nurses can be very helpful in identifying and discussing problems. If expert guidance and counselling is needed, it can be given by most breast clinics.

Patients who have a mastectomy can have plastic surgery designed to fashion a new breast. This may be done with a silicon implant or by bringing some muscle around from the back. The aim of such an operation is to give a woman a cleavage. Despite the skill of plastic surgeons there are always scars and the new breast is never the same as the original breast. It is always worth asking what can be achieved if you have had a mastectomy.

Breast conserving operations

Surgery to preserve the shape and appearance of the breast is now available. It is called a lumpectomy or quadrantectomy and removes some of the tissue around the cancer but leaves the majority of the normal breast. Such an operation is followed by radiation therapy to the remaining breast tissue to kill any cancer cells that may have been left behind. Cosmetic results can be good if patients are selected carefully; the operation is most successful if the lump is small and the normal breast is of at least moderate size.

Many doctors will not recommend this type of operation and the degree of conflict surrounding breast preservation is shown by the ruling in several American states that patients *must* be offered this option. Recent evidence has given strong support to such an approach and many surgeons are considering it for appropriate patients. There is no doubt that in selected patients it allows the normal breast to be preserved and results as good as conventional surgery have been reported when patients are selected carefully. Many surgeons, in addition to the removal of the cancer, remove lymph nodes from under the arm using the same or a separate incision. This will not lessen the cosmetic effect and is useful in helping to decide if any further treatment is necessary (see section on chemotherapy, page 125).

This type of surgical approach *together* with radiotherapy is a valid alternative to a mastectomy in selected patients and, if you have breast cancer, discuss the advantages and disadvantages with your doctor. Lumpectomy without radiotherapy is unacceptable.

Radiotherapy (Chapter 11)

After a conventional mastectomy, many patients in the past received radiotherapy to the area of the breast and its local lymph nodes. This reduces the risk of the cancer recurring locally but has no effect on the survival of patients. Recently many radiotherapists have felt that routine post-operative radiotherapy is not justified though this remains controversial. When cancer starts in the inner (medial) side of the breast radiotherapy is still used by many hospitals. Discuss the advantages and disadvantages of post-operative radiotherapy if such therapy is suggested. Radiotherapy to the remaining normal breast is usually routine for women having lumpectomy or other operations designed to conserve the breast.

• If radiotherapy is to be given, the first visit to the department is spent 'planning' the treatment. This consists of designing a personal treatment programme that is suited to the individual patient. When treatment starts it is usually given for 4 or 5 days each week and will last about 4 or 5 weeks. Because of the type of treatment given and the particular shape of the chest there may be some soreness of the skin for a short period.

• If a tumour is large when a patient first sees her doctor or if the skin of the breast is involved it is often not useful to perform a mastectomy and X-ray therapy alone may be used. This treatment may include the use of radioactive wires (implanted during an operation under anaesthetic—page 78) for a few days. Such treatment may vary considerably from patient to patient and it is worth discussing with your radiotherapist.

Hormone therapy (Chapter 12)

- Hormone therapy has been used to treat breast cancer since the last century. It was originally shown that surgical removal of the ovaries (oophorectomy) caused shrinkage of breast cancer in about one-third of patients. Since then removal of the ovaries has been the standard first-line treatment if breast cancer recurs in women before their menopause. Around one-half of patients have tumours whose growth is partly controlled by hormones and these are the ones that regress when the ovaries (which produces the hormone oestrogen) are removed. In the past few years it has become possible to identify the patients whose tumours are hormonally responsive. Tissue removed from the cancer is examined in the laboratory and levels of 'receptors' for oestrogen and progesterone can be measured. If these 'receptors' are present, over two-thirds of the patients respond to removal of the ovaries; if they are absent virtually none respond.

- Although removal of the ovaries has long been regarded as the best initial treatment for recurrent breast cancer by many doctors, new drug treatments can have similar effects. Hormone drug treatments have been used for many years, but have had side-effects that have limited their use. Tamoxifen is a drug that blocks the effects of oestrogen (produced in the ovary) and it is probably as effective as removing the ovaries. It has few side-effects and many doctors now use it instead of an operation to remove the ovaries. The advantage of avoiding an operation is obvious, especially when it is remembered that many patients may not respond to the operation. Hormone receptors are frequently measured on tissue taken at the original mastectomy and the results can be used to predict if a patient will respond to hormonal treatment later. The chances that a tumour will respond can be improved from 30 per cent to between 60 per cent and 80 per cent if patients are selected according to the receptor information.

- Patients who have responded well to one hormonal treatment are also likely to respond to different hormone therapy if the tumour grows back. This hormonal treatment may be totally different to the first one, but it seems that it is the change of the hormones in the tumour that slows its growth—indeed just stopping one hormonal treatment may cause shrinkage in the size of tumour.

Tamoxifen works by blocking the normal female hormone, oestrogen; other hormonal drugs that may be used include oestrogen-like drugs, progesterones and androgens (male hormones). Oestrogens may cause vaginal bleeding, retention of fluid, and clotting in veins. Androgens often induce changes in the body so that it becomes more male in appearance (virilization); the voice deepens and facial hair may grow. Both of these types of drug have been used extensively but their side-effects are a real problem and since the introduction of tamoxifen they are only used when other hormonal treatments have stopped working. Drugs which stop the adrenal glands working normally are also used. These glands produce a variety of hormones including cortisone. Aminoglutethimide, a drug which stops the adrenal producing female and other hormones, is always given together with prednisone (cortisone) tablets. Aminoglutethamide often causes temporary skin rashes or sleepiness, but if the tablets are continued these effects wear off and the dose can gradually be increased over 3–6 weeks.

In the past, patients who have responded to removal of the ovaries have been shown to respond to removal of the adrenals (adrenalectomy) or pituitary gland. Some patients who responded to oophorectomy have a second response to adrenalectomy and then a third response to removal of the pituitary gland. This sequence of operations is now less popular and drugs are being used instead of operations. The number of possible hormonal manoeuvres (operations or drugs) is very complicated and it is important to discuss treatment that is being planned. However, for those patients who do respond to hormones, the quality of the response and its length is usually better than other types of therapy.

Chemotherapy (Chapter 12)

Chemotherapy is the use of drugs that kill cancer cells. As discussed in Chapter 12, all anticancer drugs have side effects and because of this they are often not used for the initial therapy of recurrent breast cancer (hormonal treatments are considered first unless it is known that the tumour does not contain hormone receptors. Chemotherapy may, however, be used following mastectomy when all tumour has apparently been removed; this is known as adjuvant therapy.

Adjuvant therapy

Adjuvant therapy is treatment which is given in addition to the primary removal of a cancer. About half of the patients who have an operation for breast cancer have a recurrence of breast cancer within ten years. The risk of recurrent tumour is highest in those who are found to have cancer in lymph nodes removed at mastectomy. Because of the higher risk in these patients, adjuvant drug therapy has been tested in clinical trials both in the United States and Europe.

Results, so far, suggest the following conclusions amongst patients found to have lymph nodes involved at mastectomy (node positive).

1. For women before or at their menopause there is a definite delay in tumour recurrence and a small but definite (15%) increase in the chances of survival. It should, however, be remembered, that not all of these patients were going to relapse or die of breast cancer even if they had not received adjuvant therapy.

2. In older women, past the menopause, there is also a definite delay in recurrence but there is no improvement in survival.

Trials have compared the effects of adjuvant therapy in women with a similar group of women receiving no adjuvant chemotherapy after their mastectomy. The choice of the two treatments was by chance and the groups were as large as possible to ensure that any differences in rates of tumour recurrence or survival were due to treatment and not a fortuitous finding. All trials show some benefit for younger patients receiving adjuvant chemotherapy. Even though this benefit is not *definitely* proven many argue that if there is any potential advantage for adjuvant therapy it should be given to all young women who are node positive. This, however, ignores the penalty paid by those receiving chemotherapy (half of whom were never destined to get recurrent cancer)—the definite side-effects of treatment. Early studies used simple tablets with relatively few side-effects but most specialists feel that combinations of drugs given by intravenous injection are more effective. The side-effects (page 86) depend on the individual drugs being used but the following are common:

(a) Nausea and possibly vomiting for some hours after treatment.
(b) Tiredness and malaise.
(c) Partial or complete hair loss (very dependent on the individual drugs used).
(d) Susceptibility to infections, bruising, or bleeding.
(e) The emotional stress of prolonged drug treatment.

Treatment programmes vary, but the drugs are often given every 2 to 3 weeks for between 6 to 12 months. Appendix A outlines the common side-effects of single drugs so that an approximate idea of the effects of a particular combination can be gained from looking up the drugs to be used.

All women with cancer in lymph nodes at mastectomy should have the opportunity to discuss adjuvant treatment with their doctors. The options are: no further treatment after mastectomy, or adjuvant chemotherapy using a drug combination. In the United States combination therapy is recommended for nearly all patients; in Europe the position is more open and many doctors do not recommend adjuvant therapy or use simple adjuvant therapy.

The arguments for adjuvant treatment are strongest in young women; for women past their menopause there is little indication for such treatment. More recently tamoxifen, a hormonal drug, has been used after surgery, as an adjuvant treatment. It delays recurrence of the disease and in one trial improved survival. It's main advantage is its nearly complete freedom from side-effects. The full results of several large trials are required before its role as an adjuvant treatment can be decided on finally.

Chemotherapy for recurrent cancer

Once breast cancer has relapsed, cure is rare; but good control of the disease for long periods can be gained. Patients who have recurrent or advanced cancer which is not responding to hormone treatment are often considered for chemotherapy. Some patterns of tumour relapse, such as involvement of the liver are best treated with drugs from the start. Many of the commonly used anticancer drugs are active in breast cancer. They are often used in a combination for best effect and will be given for at least two to three courses of treatment to test their effectiveness. A decision to continue treatment (if it is effective) or to change to an alternative treatment is then made and chemotherapy will often be continued for as long as there is evidence of a continued shrinkage of the cancer. Although many drugs are moderately effective, it is rare for drug therapy to be curative, though regression of cancer may occur for long periods. Unfortunately, chemotherapy is associated with side-effects and these are shown in Appendix A.

Patients with advanced or recurrent breast cancer can often live for many years with disease. They may require treatment intermittently (with hormones or chemotherapy) during this time but some patients (especially the elderly) have very slow growing tumours that require little or no treatment.

SUMMARY OF BREAST CANCER TREATMENT

The treatment of breast cancer is very complicated. It is impossible to cover it adequately in one chapter and it is essential that patients discuss their treatment with experienced clinicians. Some guidelines can be given.

(1) All patients with a breast lump should see a doctor.
(2) A biopsy is always needed to make the diagnosis. All suspicious lumps should be biopsied, *most* are not cancer. The type of cancer operation should be discussed with the surgeon and if a limited operation is done it should usually be followed by radiotherapy.
(3) The behaviour of the tumour is influenced by the findings at operation. (a) The microscopic appearance may indicate a good outlook. (b) Involvement of the lymph nodes under the arm indicates an increased risk of tumour recurrence. (c) The presence of hormone receptors suggests a high likelihood of response to hormone treatment.
(4) Radiotherapy after mastectomy is often used for cancers

of the inner or medial part of the breast but its role in the treatment of cancers of the outer part of the breast is less clearly defined.

(5) Adjuvant chemotherapy may be used in patients with lymph nodes that are involved. A good case can be made for this treatment in young women (before or at menopause) with positive nodes. There is no case for adjuvant treatment in older women. Tamoxifen can also be used as an adjuvant treatment.

(6) Hormone therapy is usually the first treatment used when breast cancer recurs.

(7) Patients who respond to one form of hormonal treatment are likely to respond to other hormonal therapies.

(8) When tumour has recurred it is rare for cure to result from treatment and if the disease comes back after a response it is common to change to alternative treatments, either more hormones or chemotherapy.

(9) There are many active drugs in breast cancer; they are usually used in a combination.

(10) X-ray therapy is often very useful for controlling symptoms (especially pain) from recurrent cancer.

(11) Despite our inability to cure advanced breast cancer many patients survive long periods with or without treatment.

(12) Women with breast cancer need help to adjust to the situation. This help should come from family, the clinic, and if necessary from voluntary groups such as mastectomy associations.

CHAPTER 19

Cancer of the ováry

Cancer of the ovary is less common than cancer of the uterus (womb) or cervix but causes more deaths. This is because it often does not cause symptoms until it is far advanced. The tumour tends to spread over the surface of the abdominal organs without invading deeply. No one knows what causes this cancer and screening programmes have not been shown to be useful as the ovaries are difficult to get at.

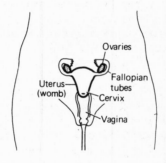

Figure 35 Diagrammatic representation of the female reproductive system showing the position of the ovaries

SYMPTOMS

Most patients present with vague symptoms and are found to have a tumour on examination. The common symptoms include:

- Abdominal discomfort or pain in the lower abdomen.
- Sudden swelling of the abdomen. This is due to the accumulation of fluid in a cyst or in the abdominal cavity (this is called ascites).
- Weight loss.

- Nausea.
- Occasionally shortness of breath due to accumulation of fluid in the chest (a pleural effusion).

DIAGNOSIS

A gynaecologist will on pelvic examination have a good idea as to whether there is a tumour in the ovary. Further tests include:

- An abdominal and pelvic ultrasound (page 45).
- Chest X-ray.
- Blood tests.
- If ascites (fluid) is present then a small needle may be passed through the skin to suck some fluid into a syringe. This fluid is examined under the microscope to see if there are any cancer cells present.

TREATMENT

The outlook and type of treatment depends very much on the stage of the tumour (Chapter 8). The extent of tumour spread is described by four stages:

Stage 1—Cancer confined to one or both ovaries.
Stage 2—Cancer has spread from the ovaries but is limited to the pelvic (or lower) part of the abdomen.
Stage 3—Cancer has spread to the rest of the abdominal organs except the liver.
Stage 4—Cancer has spread outside the abdomen or involves the liver.

The likelihood of response to treatment and outlook also depends on the appearance of the tumour under a microscope. Ovarian cancers are graded from 1 to 4 depending on their appearance; those which look most benign are grade 1 and those most malignant-looking are grade 4. Because of the influence of *stage* and *grade* the treatment of the tumour is discussed using these factor.

Stage 1

When cancer is confined to the ovaries the chance for cure is high with surgery alone.

Surgery (Chapter 10)

The essence of surgery for this tumour is a careful assessment of tumour spread and then removal of all the tumour and the local pelvic organs. If after very carefully examining the abdomen at laparotomy (an exploratory examination of the abdomen) the tumour is stage 1, then a good cancer operation includes removal of both ovaries, the fallopian tubes, and the uterus (Figure 35). The incision (cut) is usually made vertically over the lower abdomen as many surgeons do not feel that an adequate operation can be done using a bikini line incision (also known as a Pffanansteil incision). If such an operation is done the chance of cure is about 80 per cent. When the grade of the tumour is taken into account those with a good grade (1 or 2) have an even better chance of cure but those with a grade 3 or 4 tumour have less chance of cure and may be candidates for more treatment.

In young women who wish to retain their fertility the extent of surgery must be discussed very carefully. If a small tumour is confined to one ovary there may be a role for less surgery in *selected* cases. The risks must be carefully balanced and fully discussed before operation. An incomplete operation increases the risk of relapse but retains fertility. If a lesser operation is contemplated then the other apparently normal ovary should be biopsied and examined by frozen section (a technique for immediate examination under a microscope) as involvement of both ovaries is common. If all the frozen sections biopsied are clear of tumour then an operation leaving one ovary, fallopian tube, and uterus can be performed. It must be stressed, however, that such a procedure should not be used routinely and is only appropriate in carefully selected cases where young women are anxious to have children and where the tumour is very small.

Radiation therapy (Chapter 11)

No further treatment is required for those patients with a good grade (1 or 2) stage 1 tumour. For those with a poor grade (3 or 4) stage 1 tumour the chance of tumour recurrence is higher and some hospitals use radiotherapy. The best way of giving radiotherapy or chemotherapy for these patients is still unclear. In the past X-ray treatment was only given to the lower abdomen (pelvis) and tumour relapses occurred in the upper abdomen. For this reason many modern radiotherapy centres give radiation to the whole abdomen and pelvis. This treatment is very much more extensive but successfully stops tumour recurrence in the upper abdomen.

The first visit to radiotherapy is spent planning the individual treatment and patients should discuss the type of treatment to be given and its side-effects (Chapter 11). Treatment is usually given for 4 or 5 days each week and if the pelvis alone is treated it takes 3–4 weeks. If the abdomen and pelvis are treated the time taken is 6–8 weeks. Various special methods of treating the abdomen exist and these should be discussed with the patient.

The major side-effects are:

- Nausea and vomiting, especially when treating the abdomen.
- Loss of appetite.
- Tiredness.
- Diarrhoea, especially when treating the lower abdomen or pelvis.

Chemotherapy (Chapter 12)

Although a number of drugs are available for ovarian cancer they do not have an established role in treating early tumours. Some doctors are using anticancer drugs after surgery to try to improve the results—this treatment is experimental at present.

Stage 2

If it is possible to remove all evidence of tumour, survival is good. Tumour grade also reflects the likelihood of response and survival.

Surgery (Chapter 10)

The aim is removal of all tumour, both ovaries, fallopian tubes, and uterus (abbreviated to BSO and TAH). If this cannot be done as much tumour as possible is removed (known as debulking). Operations to preserve fertility have no role if the cancer involves other organs in the pelvis.

Radiotherapy

In patients who have had a complete removal of tumour, radiotherapy to the pelvis or abdomen (see stage 1) is used by some centres. If minimal tumour (this may not be visible) is left after operation (BSO and TAH) the chances of cure are high (60 per cent or more) when radiotherapy is used after surgery. When a complete operation is not possible and a greater bulk of tumour is left behind radiotherapy is less useful.

Chemotherapy

Chemotherapy is not used routinely in patients who have a complete operation (BSO and TAH) as radiotherapy is effective. In patients who have large amounts of tumour left after an operation for stage 2 ovarian cancer, chemotherapy is given in the same way as for patients with stage 3 or 4 cancer (see next section).

Stage 3 or 4

Unfortunately the chances of a cure in advanced ovarian cancer are not good (in the past less than 10 per cent of patients survived five years) but surgery remains important and the main aim is to remove as much cancer as possible.

Surgery

Even when cancer appears widely spread it is sometimes technically possible to remove all or nearly all visible cancer. This is because the tumour does not invade deeply into tissues and the cancer and organs to be removed can often be separated from the normal structures to be left behind. Ideally the operation should include removal of all tumour masses, the ovaries, fallopian tubes, uterus and omentum (a large fatty sheet in the abdomen which is a common site of tumour spread). If this type of operation cannot be done then an attempt to remove as much tumour as possible is made. The least that should be done is to take a biopsy (sample of tissue) to confirm the diagnosis.

Radiation therapy

In stage 3 tumours, when a complete operation has been done and there is minimal tumour remaining, some hospitals use radiotherapy. This should be given to both the abdomen and pelvis (see treatment of stage 1 and 2) and results with selected patients in some centres have been encouraging. Radiation has no place in the treatment of patients who have a lot of tumour after operation or who have a stage 4 cancer.

Chemotherapy (Chapter 12)

For the past 20–30 years alkylating agents (see Chapter 12 and Appendix A) have been the first choice in the treatment of stage 3 or 4 ovarian cancer. About one-half of patients treated with these drugs have a useful response to treatment. Side-effects of these drugs, which are given by mouth, are usually few. They may be given continuously or for several weeks each month. Cures with these treatment are very uncommon and the treatment is usually continued for several years or till the cancer relapses.

More recently drugs have been used in combination with better results in the short term. Such treatment is still being evaluated but of course produces many more side-effects.

The drugs commonly used (see Appendix A) are:

- Adriamycin.
- Cyclophosphamide.
- Chlorambucil.
- Cisplatin.
- Hexamethylmelamine.
- 5-Fluorouracil.
- Methotrexate.

A number of combinations of these drugs have been used but no ideal combination has been found. A rough idea of the side-effects of a particular combination can be gained from looking up the individual drugs in Appendix A. Combinations are more effective at reducing the size of a tumour but it is not clear whether long term remissions or cures are going to result. This type of chemotherapy is usually given intermittently (every 3–4 weeks) for a variable number of cycles (usually 6 or more) and if after several treatments the tumour is not responding the chemotherapy should be changed. At the end of the drug treatment if there is no evidence of a tumour a second operation may be considered. At present, second laparotomies (an exploratory operation) are being done more frequently but they have no proven value. The *possible* advantages are: (a) they allow greater certainty in the decision to stop what may be unpleasant treatment if no tumour is found and (b) if tumour is discovered this may have become surgically removable and the operation can then be followed by more chemotherapy.

SUMMARY OF THE TREATMENT OF OVARIAN CANCER

(1) No predisposing cause is known and screening is of no use.
(2) Over half of all patients have advanced disease when first seen.
(3) Response to treatment and the chances of survival are related to the spread of the cancer (stage) and its appearance under the microscope (grade).
(4) Survival is good with surgery alone in stage 1 and further treatment is only indicated in patients with a poor grade tumour. Abdominal and pelvic radiotherapy may be given to these patients. Operations preserving fertility should be planned very carefully and are only appropriate in specially selected cases.
(5) Survival is moderately good in stage 2 disease. Surgery is the main stay of initial treatment. If a complete operation has been done, abdominal and pelvic radiotherapy is given. If surgery is incomplete then chemotherapy is indicated.
(6) For stage 3 and 4 tumours surgery is still important and the aim is to remove as much tumour as possible. If a complete operation for stage 3 is done, radiotherapy to the abdomen and pelvis may be used. Other patients should receive chemotherapy. This may be simple treatment (an alkylating agent—Appendix A) which is moderately effective and has few side-effects. Alternatively a combination of drugs can

be used; these cause more side-effects but are better at reducing the size of a tumour and *may* allow a longer remission. These two types of treatment are being tested in trials and it is worth discussing the options with your doctor as no-one yet knows which is best.

(7) Second-look laparotomies are operations used to see if there is any remaining tumour at the end of treatment (usually chemotherapy). They are designed to: (a) allow the doctor to be as certain as possible that all the cancer has been destroyed before he or she stops treatment and (b) give a chance to remove any remaining tumour. No trials have tested if a second operation changes a patient's chance of survival and patients should discuss the advisability of a 'second-look' with their surgeon.

CHAPTER 20

Cancer of the uterus (womb)

Because the lining of the uterus (Figure 36) is known as the endometrium, cancer of the uterus is often called endometrial cancer. The most common tumours of the uterus are not cancer at all, they are *benign* tumours called fibroids. These may cause excessive bleeding during menstrual periods (menorrhagia) or discomfort and this may be treated with a hysterectomy (surgical removal of the uterus). If fibroids are found no further treatment is needed as they are entirely harmless.

Cancers of the uterus usually develop later in life than fibroids. They are most common in women who are over-weight, have no children, have had a late menopause and have received long-term oestrogen drug therapy.

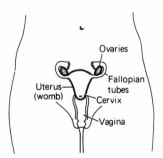

Figure 36 Diagrammatic representation of the female reproductive system showing the position of the uterus (womb)

Screening programmes have not been useful. Although a cervical smear (page 59) may pick up cancer of the uterus, it is not very helpful as it only tends to be positive in advanced cases.

SYMPTOMS

The most common symptom of cancer of the uterus is abnormal vaginal bleeding. This may be a change in periods if a woman is still menstruating and if you have bleeding between periods or after intercourse seek advice from your doctor. Similarly all women who have vaginal bleeding after their periods have stopped at the menopause should see their doctor. In most cases there is an innocent reason for the bleeding but the only way to be sure is to check.

Other symptoms may include abdominal discomfort or an offensive vaginal discharge.

DIAGNOSIS

A minor operation known as a D and C, where the lining of the womb is scraped away for examination, is the usual way of diagnosing this type of cancer (page 20). This operation is done for many different reasons and it does not mean that cancer is present. Recently a new technique using an injection of a jet spray of fluid into the uterus has been introduced. It dislodges cells from the lining and these are collected and examined under a microscope. It is not available in most centres and a D and C is a more certain way of making the diagnosis.

If cancer is found the following tests are often done before surgery.

- Chest X-ray.
- Intravenous pyelogram (IVP, page 34).
- Blood tests.
- Abdominal ultrasound (page 45) or CT scan (page 47).

TREATMENT

The usual treatment is surgery to remove the tumour. Radiotherapy and hormonal therapy are also important.

Surgery (Chapter 10)

Before the operation begins the surgeon will carefully assess the extent of tumour spread. In addition to the tests above he will perform a careful pelvic (vaginal) examination under anaesthesia (known as an EUA). When the muscles are relaxed it is possible to get a much better idea of the size and spread of the cancer.

If the tumour is confined to the uterus and has not spread deeply into its muscular wall it is curable in about 90 per cent of cases by an operation removing the uterus and ovaries (a hysterectomy and bilateral salpingo-oophorectomy). An incision (cut) is made into the lower abdomen. Most patients should be up and about the day after the operation and are usually discharged after around 10 days. Full recovery from the operation may take several months.

If the cancer is deeply invading the muscular wall of the uterus, then radiation therapy and surgery are often used together. The best treatment is probably radiotherapy given externally and internally with radiation implants (see Chapter 11) and an operation to remove the uterus and fallopian tubes. It is important to discuss the type of radiotherapy and the timing of surgery before treatment starts, as each treatment is arranged for the individual patient. About half of the patients treated in this way are cured.

Radiotherapy (Chapter 11)

When cancer has spread outside the uterus and is involving the organs in the lower abdomen, surgery has no part in treatment. Radiotherapy (given 4–5 times a week for about 4 weeks with or without radiation implants, Chapter 11) is used and can provide good control of the cancer and its symptoms. The chance of cure is small (about 10 per cent), and is best in those with the least amount of cancer.

Hormonal therapy

Hormonal therapy is used in patients with very advanced tumours or those who have recurrent tumour after surgery or radiotherapy. Progesterone, a female hormone, is helpful in about 30 per cent of cases and for those who respond the effect can last for a considerable time. The major side-effects of progesterone are occasional nausea and development of fluid retention (this may cause swelling of the ankles and legs, and if severe, shortness of breath).

Chemotherapy (Chapter 12)

Although there are some useful drugs available for this cancer only a few patients have a good response to treatment. Because of this, drug therapy of cancer of the uterus is best reserved for patients being treated in trials.

SUMMARY OF TREATMENT OF CANCER OF THE UTERUS

(1) The use of long-term oestrogen therapy can increase the risk of this cancer.
(2) Early diagnosis is difficult and screening is of no use.
(3) Any woman with vaginal bleeding between periods or after the menopause should see her doctor immediately.
(4) A small operation called a D and C is needed to make the diagnosis.
(5) Surgery cures nearly all cases.
(6) When the cancer is widely spread in the muscular wall of the uterus, radiotherapy and surgery is necessary. About half of the patients will be cured.
(7) If the cancer has spread beyond the uterus few patients are cured and radiotherapy is used.
(8) Hormone therapy is very useful in about one-third of patients.
(9) Chemotherapy is only experimental.

CHAPTER 21

Cancer of the cervix (neck of womb)

Cancer of the cervix (Figure 37) is one of the few tumours where screening to detect early cancer is routinely used and has a definite role. Despite this, there is no general agreement as to when screening should start or how often it should be done. The subject is discussed more fully in Chapter 5. Cervical cancer is most common in women who start having sexual intercourse at an early age and with many men. Virus infections that can be transmitted during intercourse have been linked with cervical cancer though the evidence is not conclusive. Cervical cancer is less common in women married to circumcised men.

Unfortunately women at highest risk are less likely to have routine screening pelvic examinations and cervical smears (page 12). This is very important as the current management of cervical cancer is largely based on early diagnosis by smear. In addition to detecting cancer of the cervix, they can recognize abnormal cells (known as dysplastic cells) which may develop into cancer (pre-malignant changes). Women with these changes

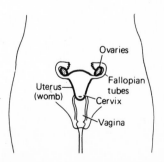

Figure 37 Diagrammatic representation of the female reproductive system showing the position of the cervix (neck of the womb)

should be watched very closely. Many do *not* go on to develop a cancer but some will.

SYMPTOMS

Ideally the diagnosis should be made by screening before symptoms appear, because by the time there are symptoms the tumour is often already advanced. Symptoms include:

- Offensive vaginal discharge.
- Bleeding between periods or after sex.
- Late symptoms may include lower abdominal pain or difficulty in passing urine.

DIAGNOSIS

There is rarely difficulty in diagnosing this tumour as the cervix can be easily seen and felt during a pelvic examination and a sample of the surface of the cervix taken by a smear.

If cancer is found the following tests may be done:

- Chest X-ray.
- Routine blood tests.
- Intravenous pyelogram (IVP, page 34).
- Pelvic ultrasound (page 45) or CT scan (page 47).
- Lymphangiogram (page 38).
- An examination under anaesthesia (EUA) is carried out to estimate the extent of spread. This is done immediately before any operation, as the pelvic muscles are then relaxed.

TREATMENT

The management of cervical cancer in the early stages depends on the cervical smear findings and stage (page 26). If cancer is suspected on the smear, a biopsy is indicated. This may be by colposcopy (examination of the cervix using a magnifying instrument) or by a cone biopsy, where a ring of the surface of the cervix is removed.

Surgery (Chapter 10)

If on cervical smear and biopsy the tumour is confined to the surface of the cervix it is called an *in situ* cancer or stage 0. Ideally the treatment of a stage 0 cervical cancer is removal of the cervix and uterus (a hysterectomy); this is curative in nearly all cases. In young women who wish to have children a cone biopsy alone may be done and further surgery delayed till after she has had children. This approach can only be used if *regular* check-ups are done to look for recurrence of the cancer.

Following a hysterectomy patients are up the next day and are ready to leave hospital at about 10 days though it takes 2–3 months to get back to normal. The incision (cut) is made over the lower abdomen.

- If the tumour has invaded the cervix itself it is called a Stage 1 tumour. Both surgery and radiotherapy can be used to treat this stage and most of the women will be cured. The main problem with surgery is the risk of complications. The commonest of these are wound and urinary infections or more seriously, although rare, are holes (fistulae) developing between the vagina and rectum. Radiotherapy also causes side-effects: thickening of the tissues is common, with dryness of the vagina, and, rarely fistulae develops. Complications are most common when surgery and radiotherapy are used together. Treatment should be planned following discussion with a surgeon and a radiotherapist.
- When the cancer has spread beyond the cervix (stages 2–4, representing increasing spread) surgery plays no role and radiotherapy is the best treatment.

Radiotherapy (Chapter 11)

Radiotherapy can be used in stage 1 cervical cancer and is always used in patients with stage 2–4 cancer. Treatment is usually given by a combination of external and internal treatment (Chapter 11), the radiation implants being placed in the uterus under anaesthesia. They are left in place for several days and then removed. The planning of radiotherapy is individualized and should be fully discussed before treatment starts. Implants are used as they deliver a very high dose of radiotherapy to the immediate area around the tumour.

Radiotherapy causes side-effects which include:

- Infertility and early menopause.
- Scarring and drying of the vagina that may interfere with intercourse (KY jelly can help).
- Diarrhoea during the treatment.
- Irritation of the bladder causing cystitis.
- Unusual late complications can include holes (fistulae) between the vagina and rectum, or bladder, and strictures (scarring and narrowing) in the rectum or bladder.

Chemotherapy (Chapter 12)

Chemotherapy is not very effective for this tumour and is not normally used except in trials testing new drugs.

SUMMARY OF THE TREATMENT OF CERVICAL CANCER

(1) Cancer of the cervix is more common in women who have had sexual intercourse at an early age and who have multiple partners.

(2) Cervical smears are an established method of screening for this tumour and have played a part in reducing the number of deaths it causes. Women with abnormal (dysplastic) cells should have regular follow-up, but many will not develop cancer.

(3) A hysterectomy is standard treatment for stage 0 cancers and is curative in nearly all cases. In young women wanting children this may be delayed if there is careful planning of treatment and follow-up screening. Stage 1 tumours may be treated by surgery alone with cure rate of about 80 per cent.

(4) Radiotherapy may also be used for stage stage 1 tumours and is as effective as surgery; it is always used for 2–4 tumours. Cure rates depend on the degree of spread outside the cervix.

(5) Sometimes surgery and radiotherapy may be used together when there is extensive disease in the cervix.

(6) Chemotherapy is experimental and not often recommended.

CHAPTER 22

Cancer of the vulva

The vulva is the external part of the female reproductive tract. Cancers are relatively uncommon at this site and usually occur late in life. No causes are known.

SYMPTOMS

These are persistent irritation, pain, or bleeding from a sore or lump on the vulva. If you have these symptoms see your doctor.

DIAGNOSIS

This is usually simple as the tumour is on the surface of the skin. A biopsy (removal of a small piece) is necessary to confirm the diagnosis.

TREATMENT

Surgery is needed and is often extensive, involving removal of the entire surface of the vulva. This is often slow to heal up, but the cure rate is high. It is worth discussing the treatment plan thoroughly before surgery.

CHAPTER 23

Cancer of the vagina

This is an unusual cancer that tends to occur in older women. In the past decade it has been seen in young women whose mothers were given oestrogens during pregnancy to try to avoid a miscarriage. Women whose mothers were known to have received hormones (usually stilboestrol) during pregnancy should have frequent screening examinations as early diagnosis is important.

SYMPTOMS

The usual symptoms are vaginal discharge or abnormal bleeding and pain.

TREATMENT

Surgery is not helpful. Radiotherapy with external and internal implant treatment (Chapter 11) is usually required. The chances of cure are related to the degree of spread of the cancer. About one-third of all patients are cured.

CHAPTER 24

Choriocarcinoma

This is a rare cancer of the placenta (afterbirth). The placenta is the organ that links a baby's blood circulation with that of its mother; it is important in supplying oxygen and nutrients. The tumour only develops in about one in every 40,000 pregnancies.

About half of the cases of choriocarcinoma develop from an abnormality of the placenta called a hydatidiform mole. This is not a cancer itself and is uncommon (1 in 2000 pregnancies) but occasionally it may progress to a malignant tumour. All patients with a 'mole' should have very close follow-up to detect any change indicating cancer.

A choriocarcinoma may develop after a normal pregnancy or a miscarriage or abortion. One of the main characteristics of this tumour is its early invasion into blood vessels and very rapid spread through the body.

SYMPTOMS

These may be from a tumour in the uterus (womb) or from distant spread of the tumour.
- Continued vaginal bleeding after the birth.
- Abdominal pain.
- Cough caused by tumour spread to the lungs.
- Neurological symptoms because of spread to the brain.

DIAGNOSIS

This includes assessment of the local tumour and any spread that may have occurred already. This tumour always produces a marker protein which can be measured in the blood. Human chorionic gonadotrophin, HCG for short, which is produced by the placentra during pregnancy, is also made by this tumour. It is useful for making the diagnosis and following the tumour's response to treatment.

TREATMENT

Although it is a tumour that spreads rapidly, most cases can be *cured* by chemotherapy (Chapter 12). Surgery and radiotherapy are usually not required.

This is a rare cancer and its treatment is very specialized and needs to be carefully planned according to the level of HCG in the blood. In most industrialized countries there are centres that specialize in the treatment of this tumour and **all** patients should go to one of these centres. This is a curable tumour and the best chance for cure lies in expert treatment.

Methotrexate (Appendix A) has been the mainstay of treatment but other drugs are also used. Even when tumour has spread to the brain patients can be cured.

CHAPTER 25

Kidney cancer

Kidney cancer, though relatively uncommon, is seen rather more often in men and usually occurs after the age of 50 years. Some of the chemicals used in industry can cause this tumour and smoking is known to increase the risk of kidney cancer by about five times. It is sometimes called renal cell carcinoma or hypernephroma. The anatomy of the urinary system is shown in Figure 38.

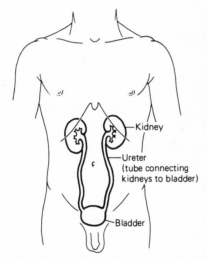

Figure 38 Diagrammatic representation of the urogenital system showing the position of the kidneys

SYMPTOMS

Often symptoms do not appear until the tumour is well advanced. The majority of patients develop symptoms because of local effects of the tumour, though some patients notice more a general illness first.

The common symptoms are:

- Blood in the urine.
- Pain in the flanks.
- Tiredness and a feeling of being 'one degree under'.
- Fevers.
- Loss of appetite and weight loss.
- Because it is a tumour that spread to bone, the first sign is occasionally pain in a bone or a fracture for no obvious reason.
- Rarely, patients may develop symptoms caused by thickening of the blood. (The kidney tumour produces a hormone that tells the bone marrow to make too many red blood cells.)

DIAGNOSIS

Unless there are symptoms suggesting something wrong with a kidney, diagnosis can be tricky. On examination it may be possible to feel a lump in the region of the kidney and a sample or urine may show signs of blood. If a tumour is suspected further tests must be done and include:

- An intravenous pyelogram (page 34).
- Ultrasound of the abdomen (page 45) or a CT scan (page 47).

If, from these, it seems likely that a tumour is present:

- An arteriogram (page 41) may be performed.

TREATMENT

Before deciding on treatment still further tests are needed to see if the tumour has spread. These include:

- CXR, whole lung tomograms (page 44) or CT scan of the chest (page 47).
- Venogram (page 41) to check whether the tumour is invading the main abdominal vein.
- Bone scan (page 49).
- Liver scan (page 50).

If these tests show no evidence of tumour spread there is a chance of a cure with an operation to remove the affected kidney (a nephrectomy).

Surgery (Chapter 10)

If a localized kidney cancer is removed patients have an excellent chance of cure. There is also a chance, though reduced, of complete cure in those patients who have involvement of draining lymph glands. In patients with widespread disease (metastases) a nephrectomy may be done if they are feeling well in themselves. Removal of the kidney is done to avoid local symptoms, but is not helpful in patients who are already ill because of spread of their cancer.

Radiation (Chapter 11)

Radiation can be helpful if the disease has spread to bone.

Hormones (Chapter 12)

Occasionally patients have shrinkage of their tumour when treated with progesterone or androgen hormones. These treatments are relatively free of side-effects and are probably worth trying in advanced disease.

Chemotherapy (Chapter 12)

Drugs are unhelpful in the treatment of this tumour and should be avoided. There are no useful new drugs though trials of experimental chemotherapy drugs continue.

Although the treatment of metastatic disease is poor the outlook for patients with spread is uncertain. If patients are feeling unwell because of their tumour, survival is not good; but some patients who have few general symptoms do quite well, despite continued metastatic disease. Very rarely this extensive disease may disappear; this is known as a 'spontaneous regression'. It is said to be more common if the kidney tumour is removed and has been used as a reason for operating on patients with widespread disease. Nephrectomy in this situation should only be done on those who are generally well and the main reason for the operation is to prevent local symptoms.

SUMMARY OF THE TREATMENT OF KIDNEY CANCER

(1) Certain chemicals are known to cause kidney cancer.
(2) Smoking increases the risk.
(3) Most patients develop local symptoms though about one-third only have general complaints.
(4) If the tumour is confined to the kidney most people are cured by its removal.
(5) Treatment for disease that has spread is poor though radiotherapy may be useful for bone spread. Chemotherapy should not be used. Hormonal therapy is relatively simple but is only useful in a few patients.
(6) Despite widespread metastatic disease the outlook is variable and occasionally patients survive years with cancer. Very rarely a spontaneous regression will occur.

CHAPTER 26

Bladder cancer

This is the most common tumour of the urinary tract and usually occurs in people aged between 50 and 70 years. Aniline dye and some chemicals in industry can cause this tumour which is also more common in smokers. The anatomy of the urinary system is shown in Figure 39.

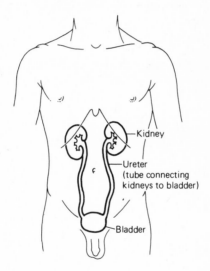

Figure 39 Diagrammatic representation of the urogenital system showing the position of the bladder

SYMPTOMS

- Blood in the urine is the first sign of cancer in three-quarters of cases. However, remember that most people with blood in their urine do not have cancer, though it is a symptom

153

which always needs investigation. Bleeding is often inter-
mittent and this should not delay investigation.
- Bladder irritability with frequency and pain on passing urine.
- In advanced cases lower abdominal pain may be a problem.

DIAGNOSIS

This is relatively easy as it is possible to look directly into the
bladder using an instrument called a cystoscope. The tests used
include:

- Microscopic examination of the urine for evidence of blood
  or infection.
- Microscopic examination of the urine looking for cancer
  cells.
- Intravenous pyelogram (page 34), an X-ray outlining the
  urinary system.
- Cystoscopy, so that the doctor can look directly into the
  bladder and can remove (biopsy) any suspicious areas.
- Under anaesthetic a careful examination of the pelvis is often
  done as the muscles are relaxed.

If a cancer is found additional tests will include:

- Chest X-ray.
- Routine blood tests.
- Possibly, a liver ultrasound (page 45) and a bone scan (page
  49).
- Some patients may also have a lymphangiogram (page 38)
  to outline the lymph nodes at the back of the abdomen.

TREATMENT

This depends on several factors. The stage of spread of the
cancer, its appearance under the microscopic (grade—the higher
the grade the more aggressive its behaviour), and its location
in the bladder. This tumour responds, up to a point, to both
surgery and radiotherapy.

Surgery (Chapter 10)

Treatment depends on the stage and grade.

- Endoscopic resection of the tumour. This means the removal of tumour whilst looking through a tube into the bladder (cytoscopy). Under anaesthetic a tube is passed into the bladder through the urethra (tube from the bladder) and this allows the doctor to examine the surface of the bladder and to remove any cancer on the lining of the bladder wall. Patients with low grade cancers of the surface of the bladder lining are treated this way. Repeat cystoscopies are required and may be needed every few months, for years in some cases.

- Segmental resection of the bladder. This is an operation to remove part of the bladder containing a single large tumour. As bladder cancers are usually widespread this is rarely done, but if it is reserved for single, large, surface tumours of low grade it can be useful.

- Total cystectomy with urinary division. This is an operation to completely remove the bladder. As the bladder has been removed, the ureters (the tubes from the kidney to the bladder—Figure 39) have to be moved so that the urine can be collected. This is a difficult procedure and there are several ways that it can be approached. Before such an operation it is *essential* all the details are discussed with the surgeon and a stoma nurse (a nurse specially trained to look after patients undergoing such surgery). The operations are:

(a) An ileal loop (page 295), which is perhaps the most common operation. The ureters are connected to part of the small bowel (the ileum) and this is brought up to the skin so that a bag can be used to collect the urine.

(b) Rectal bladder. A colostomy (page 291) is performed so that faeces are collected in a bag. The ureters are then connected to the rectum which acts as the bladder.

(c) Uretero–cutaneous. This means bringing the ureters directly up to the skin of the abdomen where a bag can be put over the stoma (the hole where the ureter is brought to the skin).

These types of operation sound quite mutilating, but if used in carefully selected patients, can be curative and work very well. Despite anxieties most patients learn to adjust to having a urinary diversion and are able to lead normal lives. The operation is probably best reserved for patients with high grade tumours invading the wall of the bladder and some cases of lower grade surface tumours which are very unresponsive to lesser treatments. An operation for urinary diversion may also be performed in patients who have widespread disease with the intention of preventing a local problem.

Radiotherapy (Chapter 11)

Once again this is complicated and includes different techniques (external and internal implant therapy—page 78), for treatment at different stages of spread and combined treatment with surgery.

Radiotherapy may be used in the following situations.

- After removal of low grade tumours of the surface of the bladder lining by cystoscopy has failed.
- When there are many large (wart-like) cancers of the bladder lining.
- When a superficial tumour changes to a high grade.
- As an alternative to removal of the bladder (cystectomy) when the patient's general health is poor.
- When simple treatment had failed to control high grade tumours that are in the bladder wall.
- Trials combining radiotherapy and surgery have been run for some years and continue.
- To provide control of symptoms such as pain or bleeding into the bladder when a tumour is widespread.

The technique of radiation is variable, but unless implants (page 78) are used, treatment is usually given for 4 or 5 days a week for 5–6 weeks. Side-effects of radiotherapy include:

(1) Discomfort and increased frequency of passing urine. These are temporary and can usually be controlled.
(2) Diarrhoea, which can also be reduced.
(3) A risk of local infection.
(4) Late complications can include prolonged inflammation of the bladder, shrinking and scarring of the bladder, bleeding from the bladder, and prolonged diarrhoea.

If implant treatment is to be used the technique will need to be discussed with the doctor as the type of treatment may vary between patients.

Chemotherapy (Chapter 12)

Although several drugs are useful for bladder cancer there is no convincing evidence that combinations of drugs are much better than each drug used alone. The major drugs are adriamycin, 5-FU, methotrexate, thiotepa and cisplatin (Appendix A). All these drugs cause side-effects and this must be borne in mind when discussing treatment. About a quarter of patients will find these drugs temporarily helpful, but the benefits must be weighed against the toxicity and because of this there is no role for combination drug treatment except in trials. An idea of the side-effects of the drugs used can be gained from looking at Appendix A. Some drugs may be used by instilling them directly into the bladder, though this is largely experimental.

SUMMARY OF THE TREATMENT OF BLADDER CANCER

(1) Some chemicals are known to cause bladder cancer and smoking increases the risk.
(2) Care of this tumour is complicated and a collaborative approach (surgery, radiotherapy, and medical oncology) is often necessary.
(3) The amount of spread of a tumour and its appearance under a microscopy (grade) are important in choosing treatment.
(4) Surgery or radiotherapy may be used separately or together.
(5) The choice of the most appropriate treatment should be tailored for each patient and needs to be discussed fully before a final decision is made.
(6) If a cystectomy (removal of the bladder) is performed a great deal of support and the advice of a stoma nurse is needed.
(7) The chances of survival depend very much on the extent of spread and the tumour grade.

CHAPTER 27

Cancer of the prostate

The prostate gland is located at the base of the bladder and is just in front of the rectum and can be felt during a rectal examination. Cancer of the prostate is common in older men and nine out of every ten cases occur after the age of sixty. The incidence increases with each year and 15 per cent or more of men over 60 years of age have the tumour, but most are slow-growing cancers of low grade malignancy that never give trouble. No cause is known.

SYMPTOMS

Because it is commonly a slow-growing tumour many men die of other causes without ever realizing that they had the cancer. In others it is an incidental finding at an operation to remove a benign enlarged prostate gland (benign prostatic hyperplasia). Some tumours are found as a hard nodule in the prostate on routine rectal examination.

Most, however, cause difficulties in passing urine.

- Increased frequency of passing urine.
- Difficulty in emptying the bladder completely.
- Getting up at night to pass urine.
- Pain on passing urine.
- Blood in the urine.

Because the tumour tends to spread to bones the first symptom may occasionally be pain in bones.

DIAGNOSIS

This tumour is diagnosed by rectal examination and then a needle biopsy (page 66). This is done under local anaesthetic, usually through the rectum, and should not be painful. Because this tumour produces a chemical called acid phosphatase, a blood test will be done to see if it is present at raised levels in the blood.

Tests to look for spread of tumour will include:

- Isotope bone scan (page 49).
- X-rays of bones suspicious on the bone scan.
- Intravenous pyelogram (IVP, page 34).
- Occasionally, a lymphangiogram (page 38) to look at the abdominal lymph nodes.

TREATMENT

The choice of treatment depends on age, the extent of the disease and the patient's general condition. The options are surgical removal of the gland, radiation, or hormonal treatments.

Surgery (Chapter 10)

This is used in younger men, in good health, who have a cancer that has not spread beyond the prostate gland. Operations often affect sexual potency and radiotherapy may be used as an alternative treatment.

Radiotherapy (Chapter 11)

When it is used in disease localized to the prostate about 50–70 per cent of patients will survive for 5 years and most will retain their sexual potency. Survival results are similar to those achieved with surgery.

If the tumour has spread outside the prostate gland, but is not involving bones, radiation is used. This may be together with limited surgery and implant radiation therapy (page 78) may be used as well as external radiation.

Hormone therapy (Chapter 12)

Growth of this cancer is affected by hormones and removal of male hormones and replacement with female hormones will slow down the tumour's growth. This may be done by removing the testicles (castration) or by giving female hormones tablets (oestrogens). Although these treatments sound drastic and affect sexual function they can give complete and prompt relief from bone pain or urinary obstruction that can last for several years. They cannot, however, cure the cancer.

Chemotherapy (Chapter 12)

Chemotherapy should only be used in trials testing new treatments as the available drugs are of very limited value.

SUMMARY OF THE TREATMENT OF PROSTATE CANCER

(1) It is common in men over 60 years.
(2) It is often a slow-growing tumour.
(3) Symptoms of difficulty in passing urine are common.
(4) The chance of cure is best when the cancer has not spread beyond the prostate gland.
(5) Surgical removal of the gland usually causes loss of sexual potency but may be curative in the early stages.
(6) Radiotherapy may be as effective and does not affect sexual potency. Radiotherapy is also used for tumours that have spread locally.
(7) Hormone therapy is used for widespread disease. Chemotherapy is not routinely used.

CHAPTER 28

Cancer of the testicle

Although they seem to be relatively uncommon testicular tumours are the commonest type of cancer in young men (15–40 years). The only known predisposing factor is failure of a testicle to descend normally into the scrotum early in life (see page 8). There is no evidence that screening is useful but any lump in a testis should be examined by a specialist—a urologist. Although many men are reluctant to see their doctor with such a lump it is important to do so as this is one of the most curable tumours.

If a cancer is suspected a biopsy (using or needle or making an incision into the scrotum) should **not** be done. This may spread the cancer; an operation, in the groin, to take out and examine the affected testis should be done and if the testis contains cancer it should be completely removed. Men who only have one testis are perfectly normal sexually and can father children.

If the testis is shown, under a microscope, to contain cancer it may be one of two types.

- Seminoma.
- Teratoma.

Because the treatment of each type is different they are discussed separately. The only common symptom of either type is a swelling (painful or painless) of a testicle. Occasionally swelling of one or both breasts may be noted.

SEMINOMA

This is commonest in the age group 30–40 years and is less 'malignant' than teratomas. They account for about half of the malignant tumours of the testis and spread from the testis to the lymph nodes in the abdomen. Occasionally it may spread further to the lymph nodes in the chest and eventually even into the lungs.

Because of this, staging investigations are done to see how extensively the tumour has spread. These include:

- Chest X-ray.
- Lymphangiogram (to look at the lymph nodes in the abdomen—page 38).
- CT scan to examine the abdomen and chest (page 47).
- Blood tests to look for the marker proteins HCG and AFP. These proteins are only normally produced by teratomas so that if they are present in abnormal quantities this suggests that the tumour contains a mixture of seminoma and teratoma. Such tumours should be treated as a teratoma.

Staging

Tumours are divided into three stages as follows:
I A tumour confined to the testis with no evidence of spread.
II A tumour that has spread to the lymph nodes in the abdomen.
III A tumour that has spread further and involves lymph nodes in the chest, or the lungs, and liver.

Treatment

A combination of two or more types of treatment may be needed.

Surgery (Chapter 10)

An operation (using an incision or cut in the groin) is performed to completely remove the abnormal testis.

Radiotherapy (Chapter 11)

If the tumour is stage I or II (as the great majority are) it is usual to give a course of radiotherapy to the lymph nodes in the abdomen. This will take about 3 weeks (treatment being given 4–5 times a week) and should not cause many side-effects though patients may notice some tiredness, or diarrhoea.

The vast majority of patients (95 per cent) are probably cured by this treatment.

Chemotherapy (Chapter 12)

Only a few patients have extensive disease (Stage III) or relapse after radiotherapy and are candidates for drug treatment. Recently chemotherapy of the same type given to patients with teratomas (page 165) has been used with very good results.

MALIGNANT TERATOMA

This tumour spreads by the lymph system in much the same way as a seminoma but can also spread via the bloodstream. The risk of involvement of the lungs is therefore greater. Nearly all these tumours produce one or both of the proteins HCG or AFP. HCG, or human chorionic gonadotrophin, is produced by the placenta in a normal pregnancy and AFP (alphafeto protein) is also produced (by cells called yolk sac cells) in normal pregnancy. Some of the primitive or embryonic cells that produce HCG or AFP are usually present in a teratoma. These proteins can be measured in the patient's blood and are very useful for monitoring the state of the disease at any time. The treatment, especially chemotherapy, of teratomas is complicated and they should preferably be cared for in a special cancer centre.

Investigations

These are designed to assess the extent of spread and will include some of the following.

- Blood tests for AFP and HCG.
- Chest X-ray.
- Whole lung tomograms (page 44) to look for small tumours or preferably
- CT scan (page 47) to examine the abdomen and chest.
- Lymphangiogram (page 38) to look at the lymph nodes at the back of the abdomen.
- Blood tests to measure liver and bone marrow function.

Staging

There are a number of different staging systems in use so that
this is a confusing area. However, the extent of spread divides
roughly into three major areas.

  I Tumour is localized to the testis and all tests are normal.

 II Tumour is involving lymph nodes in the abdomen.

III In this case the tumour has spread into lymph nodes in the
    chest, in the lungs, or into the liver.

Equally, as important as the stage is the amount of disease, or
bulk, at each involved site. The bigger a tumour the less good
the outlook is.

Treatment

This will depend on the stage.

Surgery (Chapter 10)

The testis is removed through an incision in the groin. In the
United States patients who, on investigation, are found to have
stage I or II disease (unless it is very extensive stage II) may
have a further operation. This is to surgically remove all the
lymph nodes at the back of the abdomen (a radical lym-
phadenectomy). Though this is a long and difficult procedure
patients are young and fit and tolerate it well. However, loss
of normal ejaculation during intercourse may be caused by
disturbance of some of the nerves at the back of the abdomen.
The condition is known as retrograde ejaculation and usually
means the man is infertile. In Europe and Britain such surgery
is usually avoided. The results of treatment are excellent with
surgery (95 per cent stage I and 85 per cent stage II are probably
cured).

Radiotherapy (Chapter 11)

In Europe patients with stage I or II disease are considered for
radiotherapy. If there is involvement of abdominal lymph nodes
only those with small tumours are treated. If patients are selected
carefully the results are about the same as for surgery, but

become less good if radiotherapy is given to patients with bulky teratomas. Radiotherapy does not cause retrograde ejaculation. Because of the success of chemotherapy, radiotherapy is now rarely used. Stage I patients are often watched and treated with chemotherapy if they relapse (15–20%).

Chemotherapy (Chapter 12)

Patients with extensive teratomas (bulky stage II or stage III) should be treated with chemotherapy. The most common treatment uses high doses of cisplatin, bleomycin, vinblastine or etoposide (Appendix A) and causes very many side-effects. Despite this it is very worthwhile treatment because the majority of patients can be cured. The major side-effects are:

- Tiredness.
- Nausea and vomiting with each treatment course.
- Abdominal pain after each treatment.
- Sore mouth.
- Risk of infection.
- Weight loss.
- Loss of hair.
- Pigmentation of the skin.
- Very occasionally damage to the lungs.
- Very occasionally damage to the kidneys.

Treatment is usually given over 5 days (in hospital) once every 3 weeks.

Other drug regimes using six or seven drugs are also being tested and may be as effective and are possibly less 'toxic'.

SUMMARY OF THE TREATMENT OF TESTICULAR TUMOURS

(1) Failure of the testicles to descend normally predisposes to a tumour.
(2) There are two major tumour types: (a) seminoma, (b) malignant teratoma.
(3) Testicular tumours should always be removed completely by an incision in the groin. Biopsies through the wall of the scrotum should not be done.

Seminoma

(4) They are commonest in the 30–40 age group.

(5) They spread by lymphatics.

(6) Most are localized to the testis or abdominal lymph nodes and can be cured (95 per cent) by radiotherapy.

(7) A few are more extensive or re-occur and can be treated with chemotherapy or radiotherapy, depending on where they are. Most of these can be cured.

Teratoma

(8) These are most common in the 15–30 age group.

(9) Most produce 'marker' proteins—AFP or HCG.

(10) Their treatment is complicated and is best done in a special cancer centre.

(11) In the United States patients with stage I and stage II (unless it is a very bulky tumour) have a second operation to remove the lymph nodes at the back of the abdomen. The results are excellent (95 per cent stage I and 85 per cent stage II cured).

(12) Such an operation may affect ejaculation and fertility.

(13) In Britain and Europe radiotherapy is sometimes given to patients with minimal stage II disease. Stage I patients are watched and treated with chemotherapy if they relapse (20%). The results of treatment are similar to those achieved with surgery.

(14) Patients with more extensive disease are treated with chemotherapy. Although the treatment has many side-effects the results are excellent with up to 60 per cent of patients with advanced disease being cured.

(15) Overall, the great majority of patients are curable; this is one of the most curable of all tumours despite its aggressive nature.

CHAPTER 29

Lung cancer

Lung cancer has, this century, increased in frequency more than any other tumour. There is no doubt that it is usually caused by cigarette smoking except in the case of one type, adenocarcinoma of the lung (see below). The risk of cancer is related to the number of cigarettes smoked and when someone stops smoking their risk of cancer gradually falls, after about 10 years, to that of a non-smoker. Members of families who have several relatives with lung cancer may be at even greater risk if they smoke. Screening tests have, unfortunately, not been successful.

Because the treatment of lung cancer is different for two main types, discussion in this chapter will be under two headings: (1) small cell lung cancer (oat cell), and (2) non-small cell lung cancer.

SMALL CELL LUNG CANCER (OAT CELL)

About a quarter of the cases of lung cancer are called small cell lung cancer. This is a rapidly growing cancer that quickly spreads to other parts of the body. Due in part to it's rapid growth, it is the type of lung cancer that is most responsive to drug and radiation treatment. It is also known by the name 'oat cell' lung cancer because its cells looks like small oat grains when seen through a microscope.

SYMPTOMS

Most patients have symptoms caused by the tumour in the lung, though occasionally spread of tumour may cause symptoms. The usual problems are:

- Cough, with or without blood.
- Chest infection that does not get better with antibiotics.
- Hoarseness.
- Pain in the chest.

- Lump in the chest wall or above a collar bone.
- Swelling of the veins in the neck.
- Rarely, symptoms caused by tumour spread to the brain.
- Rarely, symptoms caused by the tumour making large amounts of hormones.

DIAGNOSIS

A chest X-ray will in nearly all patients, show a suspicious shadow. Although patients will be asked to cough up sputum to see if it contains cancer cells most patients will need a bronchoscopy (page 64). In this test, the surgeon is able to look into the air passages in the lungs (bronchi) and can take a piece of tissue (a biopsy) from any possible tumour. If a lymph gland (usually it is in the neck) is enlarged this may also be biopsied. If it is not possible to make the diagnosis this way, it is occasionally necessary for a surgeon to make a small cut (incision) just above the breast bone at the base of the neck. He will then be able to use a tube to look into the chest and to biopsy any odd-looking glands; this test is known as a mediastinsocopy. These tests are used to diagnose the cancer and further tests are then needed to see if the tumour has spread. These tests will include some or all of the following:

- Bone scan (page 49) and possibly X-rays of some bones.
- Liver ultrasound (page 45) or scan (page 50).
- CT scan of the chest and abdomen (page 47).
- Bone marrow aspirate and biopsy (page 53)
- Occasionally a CT scan of the brain (page 47) or brain scan (page 49).

TREATMENT

Small cell lung cancer is a very rapidly growing tumour which is nearly always widely spread through the body by the time the diagnosis is made. Because of this, surgery to remove part or all of a lung is rarely curative. The one exception to this is the occasional patient who has a simple lump or tumour in the lung, which is well away from the heart, blood vessels, and glands in the centre of the chest. In these patients the diagnosis of small cell lung cancer is often only made when the lump is removed and about one-third of these patients are cured by the operation.

An operation is not useful in other patients and treatment is by chemotherapy and radiation.

Surgery (Chapter 10)

Surgery should be reserved for single tumour in the periphery of the lung and additional chemotherapy should be given after the operation. Patients undergoing chest surgery will have drainage tubes left in for several days after the operation but most will be up the day after the operation and are usually fit for discharge in about 2 weeks. It takes some months to get over chest surgery.

Radiotherapy (Chapter 11)

Radiation treatment suffers from the same disadvantages as surgery—it only treats the cancer in the local area the radiation is aimed at. Although it was originally used alone to try to prevent symptoms due to tumour growing in the chest it is now often used together with chemotherapy.

Chemotherapy (Chapter 12)

Treatment is given according to the extent of spread of the tumour. If the cancer is confined to one part of the chest only it is called a 'localized' tumour and if it has spread to any other part of the body it is called 'extensive'.

In each case the first treatment is chemotherapy and several drugs will be given in a combination, usually at 3-week intervals. A number of different combinations of drugs are used and it is important to discuss the details of the particular treatment before it starts. The most frequently used drugs are:

- Adriamycin
- Cyclophosphamide
- Vincristine
- Etoposide

The side-effects of these drugs are shown in Appendix A and a rough idea of the side-effects of a combination can be gained from looking up each of the drugs.

Localized disease

As well as chemotherapy these patients are often given radio-therapy. This may be started together with the drug treatment or may be delayed for several months while chemotherapy is given. Neither approach is proven to be better though there are more side-effects when the radiotherapy and chemotherapy are given together.

Radiotherapy is usually given to the tumour in the chest 4 to 5 days per week for 3 or 4 weeks. Side-effects include:

- Tiredness and lethargy, this is made worse by the chemo-therapy.
- Soreness on swallowing which is worse if the drug adri-amycin is being used.
- Mild nausea.

Radiotherapy is often given to the head to prevent spread of the tumour to the brain (see below). This will cause temporary loss of hair, if drug treatment has not already done so, and can occasionally cause poor memory and loss of concentration for a couple of months.

Depending on the way the treatment programme is designed it may stop at this point or more chemotherapy may be given. The usual period of treatment is 6 months to 1 year, though doctors are unsure of the optimum duration of therapy.

Extensive disease

The only role for radiotherapy when there is widespread disease is to treat symptoms; the most important treatment is chemo-therapy. Most patients respond quickly to drug treatment and if a patient has had no useful response to drugs after two or three treatments then it is doubtful that they will benefit from more chemotherapy. If patients are responding then treatment is continued with the intention of getting rid of all signs of tumour. Treatment is continued for up to a year, provided the cancer is under control.

Brain radiotherapy

There is, unfortunately, a high risk of spread of the cancer to the brain. Because of this it is common to give radiotherapy to the brain as part of the treatment. Radiotherapy is given 4–5 times a week for about 2 weeks and is very successful in preventing symptoms due to spread to the brain. Many patients are very frightened by the thought of cancer in the brain or such radiotherapy, but the brain is very resistant to radiotherapy and treatment successfully stops spread to the brain. Some doctors only given brain radiotherapy if the tumour is coming under control with chemotherapy.

Outlook in small cell lung cancer

This has changed in the last ten years. It used to be one of the most devastating cancers but is now very responsive to treatment. Most patients with localized disease have complete disappearance of the tumour with treatment and up to one in five of these patients *may* be cured and the rest have very useful prolongation of life. For those with extensive disease the outlook is not so good. Less than half will have a complete remission and very few will be cured. However, chemotherapy is useful for prolonging life in many patients. In the unlucky few who do not respond well to treatment, it is important to decide if it is useful to go on with further or different therapy.

NON-SMALL CELL LUNG CANCER

This is a collection of three different types of lung cancer which behave rather similarly. They are called:

(1) Squamous or epidermoid cancer.
(2) Adenocarcinoma.
(3) Large cell cancer.

They are grouped together because their pattern of treatment is different from small cell lung cancer.

They do not grow as quickly as small cell cancer and because of this are less often widespread at diagnosis.

SYMPTOMS

These are usually due to the tumour in the chest.

• Cough with or without blood.

- Chest infection that does not get better despite antibiotics.
- Hoarseness.
- Lump in the chest wall or above a collar bone.
- Swelling of the veins of the neck.
- Rarely, symptoms caused by too much calcium in the blood.

DIAGNOSIS

The same tests are used as in small cell lung cancer (page 00), though fewer tests are done to see if the tumour has spread. As surgery is the most important treatment, every effort is made to see if a tumour is small enough to be removed and to make sure there is no spread.

TREATMENT

If this type of lung cancer can be completely removed by an operation there is a chance of cure.

Surgery (Chapter 10)

The number of investigations before an operation varies from patient to patient but will include a bronchoscopy (page 168) and possibly a mediastinoscopy (a minor operation to look into the chest with a small telescope). Patients will also have lung function tests to see if their breathing can stand removal of some lung. If the tumour is apparently localized and surgically removable then the patient is checked to make sure there is no tumour spread elsewhere (page 23).

When all these tests are completed, unfortunately, fewer than half of patients have a small localized tumour that can be removed. These patients, if their general health is good, will have the tumour removed together with part (lobectomy) or whole (pneumonectomy) of the lung on that side. Provided they do not have chronic lung disease, patients can carry on pretty well as normal, despite having one lung removed.

Of those patients who have this type of operation about one in five is cured. The operation is done by a thoracic surgeon and patients will have drainage tubes in their chest for a few days after the operation. They will be up the day after surgery and will usually be ready to go home about 2 weeks later. Full recovery takes a couple of months.

Radiotherapy (Chapter 11)

Patients who have local tumour that cannot be removed and no other obvious spread of tumour may be treated with radiation. This type of treatment is best reserved for treating symptoms and is also very useful in dealing with pain caused by spread of the tumour. The frequency and length of treatment will depend on the aim of treatment and should be discussed with the radiotherapist.

Chemotherapy (Chapter 12)

Unfortunately there have been few improvements in the drug treatment of this type of lung cancer. Although some patients respond to treatment there is no evidence that the patients live much longer. For this reason chemotherapy should, preferably, only be used in trials.

SUMMARY OF THE TREATMENT OF LUNG CANCER

(1) Many cases are caused by smoking.
(2) Screening is not useful.
(3) There are two major groups (small cell lung cancer and non-small cell lung cancer).

Small cell lung cancer

(4) This tumour grows quickly and spreads rapidly.
(5) Surgery is only useful for a very few patients.
(6) Chemotherapy is the most important treatment.
(7) Radiotherapy and chemotherapy are given to patients with cancer confined to one side of the chest (localized disease).
(8) Chemotherapy alone is used for more extensive spread.
(9) Irradiation may be given to the brain to prevent spread.
(10) Most patients with localized disease have a complete remission; about one in five *may* be cured with radiotherapy/chemotherapy.

(11) Fewer than half of the patients with extensive disease have a complete remission and virtually none are cured.

(12) Many of the patients not cured have useful prolongation of life with treatment.

Non-small cell lung cancer

(13) Surgery is the most important treatment.

(14) Every effort is made to see if a patient is curable with an operation.

(15) Less than half the patients have an operation and about one in five of those who do are cured.

(16) Radiotherapy may be useful in controlling symptoms if the cancer is not curable.

(17) Chemotherapy does cause some shrinkage of tumour but does not improve survival.

CHAPTER 30

Cancer of the head and neck

This is a very complicated tumour as there are many different places a cancer can develop and each may behave differently. The tumours most commonly occur in eldery patients (more than 60 years).

Head and neck cancer includes tumours developing in the mouth, salivary glands, nose and air passages, the voice box (larynx), and throat. Because of the many types of cancer it is only possible to discuss treatment in general terms. These cancers are most common in those who smoke and drink heavily. Some patients may have a pre-malignant lesion in their mouth called leukoplakia which can turn into a cancer.

SYMPTOMS

This will of course depend on where the cancer is, but the common symptoms are:

- Nose and air passages: bloody discharge from nose, obstruction to breathing through the nose, pain in the teeth and face.
- Back of the nose (nasopharynx): difficulty breathing, lump in the neck, damage to nerves supplying parts of the head and neck.
- Mouth: swelling or ulcer that fails to heal, pain, lump in the neck.
- Back of mouth (oropharynx): pain or difficulty on swallowing, difficulty breathing, lumps in the neck, pain in the ear.
- Voice box (larynx) and surrounding tissues: hoarseness, difficulty on swallowing, difficulty breathing, lump in the neck.

DIAGNOSIS

This is usually relatively easy as most of these areas can be looked at or felt directly. Doctors need to have a very careful look around the mouth, back of the throat, and voice box. In order to look at the back of the mouth a mirror, like a dentist's, is warmed up before being put in the mouth (to stop condensation). The patient is asked to put his tongue out as far as possible and the doctor will hold the tip with a piece of gauze. He will then put the small mirror into the patient's mouth and take a look around. If necessary some local anaesthetic may be used to stop any gagging. Although, many patients are apprehensive before the examination it is quickly over and, if expertly done, is not unpleasant.

If a tumour is seen, or if a tumour is suspected in a spot where it would not be visible, then an examination and biopsy may be done under anaesthetic. Further investigation is needed if a cancer is found. This may include some of the following, depending where the tumour is:

- Chest X-ray.
- X-ray of the neck.
- Tomograms (page 44).
- Barium swallow (page 30).
- CT scanning (page 47).
- Ultrasound (page 45).
- Routine blood tests.
- Rarely, arteriograms (page 41).

TREATMENT

Surgery (Chapter 10)

Surgery of the head and neck is very specialized and should only be done by experts in this field. Any operation must be discussed fully with a specialist and the following important questions answered.

- Why is the operation necessary?
- How is the operation done?
- Are there any visible scars afterwards?
- Does the operation affect breathing, swallowing, or talking?

- What are the chances of cure and the chances of any unpleasant side-effects?
- Is any other treatment available and, if so, how good is it?

Many operations on the head and neck are very worrying and are sometimes disfiguring. However, if patients are selected carefully there is no doubt that many are cured by operations. Mutilating operations are not done nearly so often as in the past.

Radiotherapy (Chapter 11)

The type of radiotherapy that is given depends on the tumour. Implants (page 78) may be used though external irradiation is more common. Some radiotherapy is curative, such as in early laryngeal cancer, but much is reserved for treating symptoms. Recently radiotherapy and surgery have been used together. The radiation may be given before or after surgery and patients receiving treatment should discuss the plan before treatment is started.

Chemotherapy (Chapter 12)

Although several drugs can shrink head and neck cancers chemotherapy has yet to make much of an impact on treatment. It is being used in trials before surgery in an attempt to shrink a big tumour so that it can be removed. This approach is unproven and is best restricted to these trials. There is no good evidence that combinations of drugs are much better than one drug alone in the treatment of advanced cancer. Some of the drugs used may be toxic and it is important to balance this against any possible advantages in these elderly patients.

SUMMARY OF THE TREATMENT OF HEAD AND NECK CANCER

(1) It is a collection of very different tumours.
(2) They occur in an elderly age group and are more common in men.
(3) Tobacco and alcohol are the main causes.
(4) Surgery can be curative if a small tumour can be removed

completely. Some operations can be disfiguring and before any surgery all the options should be discussed.

(5) Radiotherapy can cure certain tumours and is usually less disfiguring than surgery. It is more often used to control symptoms.

(6) Surgery and radiotherapy are sometimes used together.

(7) Chemotherapy has yet to find a role, but is sometimes given to shrink a tumour before surgery or to try to control advanced disease.

CHAPTER 31

Hodgkin's disease

Hodgkin's disease is a cancer that starts in lymph glands. It is most common in young people and also in those over 50 years. In the past it was a difficult disease to treat because it was so relentless and patients wasted away and died after a year or two. It is now one of the recent success stories of cancer medicine. Despite this it is still a complicated disease and referral to a specialist centre is desirable.

SYMPTOMS

The commonest symptom is a painless swelling of a lymph node (gland). Lymph nodes are scattered throughout the body and are linked by fine lymph vessels (page 23). Their job is to filter out excess fluid and to remove bacteria or unwanted particles in the body; they also produce some of the lymphocytes (a type of white cell) that get into the blood. Lymph nodes are concentrated in certain sites: the neck, under the arms, in the chest around the heart, and along the main blood vessels in the abdomen. Although the commonest site of enlarged nodes in Hodgkin's disease is the neck, remember that most people with swollen lymph nodes do not have cancer, most glands swell in response to an infection. If lymph node swelling persists for several weeks advice from a doctor is needed.

Some patients have other general symptoms which can include:

- Drenching sweats at night. These may be accompanied by shivering (known as rigors) and hot and cold feelings.
- Loss of appetite and tiredness.
- Loss of weight.
- Severe itching all over.
- Pain in swollen glands on drinking alcohol which is a puzzling but uncommon symptom.

DIAGNOSIS

If there is persistent lymph node enlargement a biopsy (removal of the gland or a piece of it—page 52) should be done. This is often a minor procedure.

It is important that a biopsy is done by an experienced surgeon as future treatment depends on the adequacy of the biopsy. If a lymph node cancer is suspected the pathologist should be told before the operation so that tissue for any special tests may be collected properly. The interpretation of different types of cancer in lymph nodes is difficult and a pathologist (the doctor who examines the tissue under a microscope) may need to ask the opinion of a specialist in this field. Four subtypes of Hodgkin's disease are recognized by pathologists: (a) lymphocyte predominant, (b) nodular sclerosing, (c) mixed cellularity, and (d) lymphocyte depleted. Although considered important in the past, the chances of survival are not much different for each subtype when modern treatment is used.

STAGING

If the diagnosis of Hodgkin's disease is confirmed, the next step is to find out how far the disease has spread.

It tends to spread from one group of lymph nodes to another and then eventually into the blood and liver. The following tests are used first of all:

- Chest X-ray and sometimes whole lung tomograms (page 44) are done to see if there is swelling of the lymph glands in the chest and to examine the lungs.
- A lymphangiogram (page 38) to outline lymph nodes in the abdomen.
- Some hospitals may also use an ultrasound (page 45) or CT scan (page 47) to examine the abdomen.
- Bone marrow biopsy (page 53) to see if the bone marrow is affected.
- Routine blood tests.

A special staging system (Figure 40), is used for Hodgkin's disease.

Patients are divided into four stages according to the following criteria:

- *Stage 1:–* One group of lymph nodes involved, anywhere in the body.
- *Stage 2:–* More than one group of lymph nodes involved, but only if they are on the same side of the diaphragm (the muscle that divides the abdomen from the chest).
- *Stage 3:–* More than one group of lymph nodes involved, but on both sides of the diaphragm.
- *Stage 4:–* Involvement of the lungs, liver, bones, or bone marrow.

Patients are also divided into two further categories according to whether they have important symptom or not. Those without symptoms are called A and those with sweats and fever or appreciable weight loss are said to have B symptoms.

Typical patterns of disease and its staging are shown in Figure 40. Staging is important because the type of treatment and its chances of success are closely related to the stage at diagnosis.

When investigations are complete, patients are placed in the appropriate stage depending on the results. If a patient has disease falling into stage 1 or 2 or if they have stage 3 with no symptoms (3A) they may be considered for a special staging operation.

Because there is a risk of undetected Hodgkin's disease in the spleen, abdominal lymph nodes, and liver, many specialists recommend surgical exploration of the abdomen (a laparotomy). During this operation the spleen is removed and biopsies taken from many lymph nodes and the liver. A large bone marrow biopsy is taken as well.

The importance of the laparotomy is to ensure that all sites of disease are known so that radiation therapy can be planned if the Hodgkin's disease only involves lymph nodes. The spleen is removed to ensure that it is normal (if it is involved the risk of liver or bone marrow disease is much higher) and to protect the kidney from radiation. If the spleen is left and radiotherapy is given, the spleen which overlies the left kidney must be irradiated and this may cause permanent damage.

A staging laparotomy should be done by an experienced surgeon as it requires special care in examining all the possible sites of spread. In young women the ovaries should also be moved behind the uterus (womb) so that any radiotherapy does

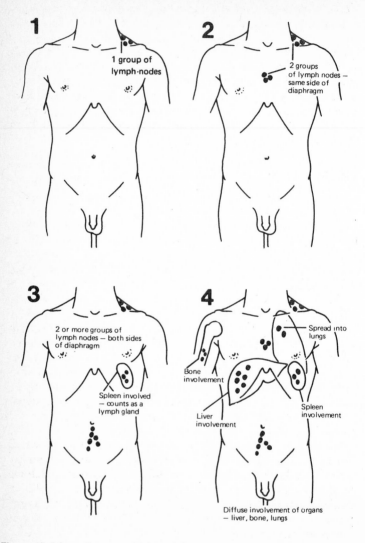

Figure 40 Schematic representation of the staging of Hodgkin's disease—see text for definition of stages

not damage them. A vertical incision over the abdomen is used and patients (who are usually young and fit) should be up the following day and be ready to go home in about 10 days.

Removal of the spleen has few effects, though children who have had a spleen removed have a higher risk of severe bacterial infections and some doctors give them long-term antibiotics or vaccines to try to prevent this. The risk in adults is much less. Some doctors do not do a laparotomy or remove the spleen in children and the pattern of treatment is usually different from that of adults (page 255).

TREATMENT

This depends on the stage of the disease after careful staging investigations.

Stages 1A to 3A

Radiation therapy is the best treatment in those patients whose disease is apparently limited to lymph nodes. The chance of cure depends on the stage and is best in those with least disease (1A) and falls off as the amount of disease increases. The great majority of patients with stage 1A are cured with radiotherapy alone, whilst about half of stage 3A patients have the tumour come back (relapse) after radiotherapy alone. However, most of those who relapse will obtain a second complete remission with drug treatment. However, because of the risk of relapse, some patients will be treated with both radiotherapy and chemotherapy. The cure rate is probably around 60–70 per cent for stage 3A.

Radiation is given to the involved lymph nodes and to all nearby lymph node areas. The overall extent of the radiotherapy depends on the amount of tumour spread. If the disease is above the diaphragm then the area or field to be treated is called a mantle (Figure 41(A)) and if the nodes are below the diaphragm a field known as an inverted Y is used (Figure 41(B)). When there is disease on both sides of the diaphragm and the patient has no symptoms (Stage 3A) radiation is given to both fields and the treatment is referred to as total nodal irradiation (TNI). In the United States TNI is often used when the lymph nodes are only involved on one side of the diaphragm.

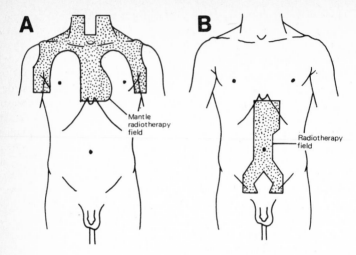

Figure 41 Schematic representation of the two common X-ray fields used for Hodgkin's disease: (a) mantle radiotherapy, (b) an inverted Y field. A radiotherapy field is the area to which the radiation is given

Radiation therapy (Chapter 11) is carefully planned and then given for 4–5 days each week for 3–5 weeks. This is the time required to treat one field (a mantle or inverted Y). If total nodal irradiation is given, then a similar period is needed for the second treatment; there is often a short gap between the two treatments.

Side-effects vary from patient to patient and include:

- General tiredness that may take 1 to 2 months to return to normal if total nodal irradiation is given.
- Soreness on swallowing during mantle radiation.
- Nausea and occasionally vomiting, especially during inverted Y irradiation.
- Reddening and irritation of the skin at the site of radiation.
- Diarrhoea during inverted Y radiotherapy.
- Cough and irritation of the lungs after mantle radiotherapy.

Discuss all the side-effects fully before treatment so that you know what to expect. The radiotherapy should be given by an experienced radiotherapist as high doses are used over large fields and careful and accurate planning is needed to get the best chance of cure with minimal side-effects. Most patients tolerate this treatment well, though radiotherapy in children has to be modified to avoid stopping bone growth. Women who receive abdominal radiotherapy (an inverted Y) can be made sterile if the ovaries are treated. Because of this, the ovaries should be moved behind the uterus (womb) at the time of staging laparotomy; this reduces the risk of infertility. In men the testes are not irradiated but should be shielded with lead during inverted Y irradiation.

Some trials using both radiotherapy and chemotherapy have been conducted to see if a combined approach is more effective. So far only very marginal advantages have been seen, and only after ten years. Because of the side-effects of this long and difficult combined treatment (see next section) it is not routinely used for all patients.

Stages 3B and 4

Radiotherapy is not used when the disease is advanced. Combinations of drugs are used for the treatment of stages 3B and 4 Hodgkin's disease (Figure 40).

There are several combinations that are commonly used. The first successful drug combination was known as MOPP and is the standard by which new treatments are judged. One of the reasons for looking for new drugs has been the side-effects of this combination. However, it is a very active treatment producing complete remissions in 70–80 per cent of cases and cure in about 40–50 per cent of patients with advanced disease.

The major side-effects of MOPP are nausea and vomiting, pins and needles and sometimes weakness in the hands and feett, thinning of hair and suppression of the bone marrow. Other regimes appear equally effective but have not been used for as long a time. These drug regimes (all made up of the first letter of the drugs used) include MVPP, chlorambucil-VPP, and ABVD. Discussion of the detailed side-effects is beyond the scope of this chapter so discuss the side-effects of chemotherapy before treatment. A rough idea of the potential toxicities can be gained from looking up the individual drugs of the particular combination in Appendix A.

The individual drugs in the combinations are:

MOPP—Nitrogen mustard, vincristine (also known as oncovin), prednisone, procarbazine.
Chlorambucil-VPP—Chlorambucil, vinblastine, prednisone, procarbazine.
MVPP—Nitrogen mustard, vinblastine, prednisone, pro-carbazine.
ABVD—Adriamycin, bleomycin, vinblastine, DTIC.

The drugs are usually injected into a vein and the treatment then repeated 1 week later. Tablets are taken with most /com-binations for 14 days after the first injection and there are rest periods of 2–4 weeks between treatments. Patients should ask for a detailed explanation of the timing (scheduling) of the drugs. If a regime that causes nausea and vomiting is used it is best to avoid driving home after treatment, though most pati-ents do not need to be admitted into a hospital for treatment. A drip or IV infusion is set up and the drugs are injected into the fluid running into the drip. Following treatment the IV infusion is taken down and patients are able to go home. Anti-sickness injections or tablets are usually given at the same time.

HODGKIN'S DISEASE THAT HAS RELAPSED

Patients whose disease returns following radiotherapy do very well with the combination chemotherapy used to treat advanced disease. For those patients who relapse after chemotherapy or who fail to respond to chemotherapy the outlook is not so good. Many will respond to further different combinations of drugs though the chance of long-term disease control is increasingly limited. In those patients who fail to have a com-plete remission with further combinations of drugs, control of the disease can often be achieved for long periods by using one anticancer drug at a time.

Such an approach is never curative but by changing the single drugs around according to the activity of the disease it is often possible to keep patients well for long periods. Some whose disease is resistant to treatment have lived with active Hodkin's disease for ten or more years where this approach is skilfully employed.

LONG-TERM EFFECTS OF TREATMENT FOR HODGKIN'S DISEASE

There are two major long-term problems.

(1) Infertility (page 91). This is a major problem in men as nearly all those receiving MOPP, MVPP, or chlorambucil-VPP combination chemotherapy are made sterile. It is claimed that ABVD (page 186) causes less sterility than the other combinations. Some women may become infertile or have an early menopause though this is less commonly a problem. Women having radiation therapy should have their ovaries moved behind their uterus at laparotomy in order to reduce the risk of infertility. The risk is greater in women older than 25 years who receive abdominal radiotherapy and chemotherapy.

(2) Second cancers. Unfortunately patients who are treated with both radiotherapy and chemotherapy are at an increased risk of developing leukaemia (page 196) or a non-Hodgkin's lymphoma (page 189). Though this risk is relatively small it is important if chemotherapy is being added to radiotherapy when the chances of cure with radiotherapy alone are high. ABVD chemotherapy is probably less likely to cause second cancers than the other types of chemotherapy.

Other long-term effects are uncommon and depend on the type of treatment given, they include scarring in the lungs and around the heart (radiotherapy), low blood counts (radiotherapy and chemotherapy), and an increased risk of severe infection after removal of the spleen.

SUMMARY OF TREATMENT OF HODGKIN'S DISEASE

(1) Hodgkin's disease is commonest in young adults; no causes are known.

(2) A biopsy of a lymph node must be taken to be sure of the diagnosis.

(3) Careful staging is necessary and may include a staging laparotomy. The presence or absence of symptoms is also important.

(4) Treatment is dictated by the extent of spread (stage).

(5) Radiotherapy is used for stages 1A to 3A. Some centres give chemotherapy and radiotherapy to selected patients.
(6) Chemotherapy using combinations of drugs, is given for patients with stages 3B and 4A and B disease.
(7) The results of treatment are good though the chance of cure is highest in those with the least extensive disease.
(8) Infertility is common in men treated with chemotherapy but is less of a problem in women.
(9) Leukaemia or non-Hodgkin's lymphoma can very occasionally follow treatment with chemotherapy and radiotherapy.

CHAPTER 32

Non-Hodgkin's lymphomas

This group of cancers arise in lymph nodes and, although they are dealt with together, they are a collection of tumours that often behave in very different ways. The conditions are separated from Hodgkin's disease (another lymph node cancer): they can be recognized as being different microscopically and in their behaviour and response to treatment. Most non-Hodgkin's lymphomas occur in people over 50 years of age though some varieties are also seen in children. No cause is known.

SYMPTOMS

The commonest symptom is a painless swelling (usually in a lymph node) which may have been present for some time and which may fluctuate in size. Often lots of lymph nodes can be felt but, unlike Hodgkin's disease (page 179), disease outside the lymph nodes (*extra-nodal disease*) is relatively common. Other general symptoms that can occur include:

- Tiredness or a general feeling of illness.
- Loss of weight.
- Fevers or profuse sweating.
- Indigestion or abdominal pain if the lymph tissue in the stomach or bowel is involved.
- Pain in the left side and abdomen from an enlarged spleen.
- Lumps in the skin or itching if the lymph tissue in the skin is involved.

DIAGNOSIS

As with all cancers the diagnosis is made by taking a biopsy (removal of all or a piece of tumour). This can often be done as an out-patient procedure though it will depend on the site of the biopsy.

When the diagnosis has been established the following tests are used to stage the lymphoma.

(1) Chest X-ray.
(2) Lymphangiogram (page 38) to look for enlarged lymph nodes in the abdomen.
(3) An abdominal ultrasound (page 45) or a CT scan (page 47) may be used to examine the abdomen.
(4) Blood and urine tests.
(5) Bone marrow biopsy and aspirate (page 53).

A staging laparotomy (page 181) is not routinely used in the non-Hodgkin's lymphomas, though some intestinal lymphomas may only be diagnosed at an abdominal operation. The staging system used is the same one developed for Hodgkin's disease (page 180).

TYPES OF LYMPHOMA

Pathologists and doctors do not know enough about the non-Hodgkin's lymphomas to allow agreement on a way of dividing lymphomas into various types. There are at present six or seven different classifications that try to do this. Although these classifications are based on different theories they all agree that non-Hodgkin's lymphomas can be divided into two broad categories.

Indolent lymphomas (also referred to as nodular lymphomas)

These lymphomas are often widespread at diagnosis (over half of all patients have involvement of the bone marrow). Most of them, when examined under a microscope, have what is described as a nodular pattern. They respond well to treatment with radiation or drugs but the disease is rarely eradicated. Even if treatment is not started straight away the outlook is quite good (most patients survive five or more years). During the course of the disease up to a quarter of patients will have a change of the lymphoma into an aggressive type.

Aggressive lymphomas (also known as diffuse lymphomas)

These are usually less widespread at diagnosis but grow more quickly and if left untreated are rapidly fatal. Some types respond well to treatment and there is a good chance of cure though this depends on the type of aggressive lymphoma and its stage at diagnosis. The chance of involvement of the tissues (meninges) around the brain is higher with some types of aggressive lymphomas.

TREATMENT

Because of the different behaviour of the two categories of lymphoma their treatment will be described separately. Treatment also depends on the stage (page 181) before treatment.

Indolent lymphomas

Stage 1

These are routinely treated with radiotherapy. The radiation field includes the known disease and nearby nodes and is not as extensive as that used for Hodgkin's disease (page 183). Unfortunately less than one in ten patients has stage 1 disease that may be cured by radiotherapy.

Stages 2 to 4

As these tumours are slow growing some doctors only treat patients with extensive disease if they are symptomatic or if the lymphoma is likely to damage an important part of the body. If this policy is followed some patients may not need treatment for long periods (up to ten years), though the number of patients needing treatment gradually increases with time. By about four years roughly half of the patients will have needed some treatment.

Both chemotherapy and radiotherapy are used and about threequarters of patients have a complete remission (page 259) with treatment. It makes little difference if the treatment is simple (local radiotherapy or a single drug) or complicated (combination chemotherapy—page 80, or chemotherapy and radiotherapy). It is therefore usually best to give a simple treatment with minimal side-effects unless a rapid shrinkage of tumour is required.

Though most patients have a complete remission the lymphoma usually comes back after a variable period (months to years). It is very unusual to get rid of the tumour competely and the idea of treatment is to keep the disease under control and the patient well. Survival is usually longer than seven years and patients may live for ten to twenty years.

Some patients have a change in the character of their lymphoma from a slow-growing or indolent to an aggressive type. If this occurs they should be treated as for the aggressive lymphoma, and if they have not had previous drug treatment they stand a reasonable chance of a complete remission.

When chemotherapy is used for indolent lymphomas a single drug—often cyclophosphamide or chlorambucil (Appendix A)—is usually adequate. In some cases a combination of drugs may be used, the commonest of which is known as CVP (cyclophosphamide, vincristine and prednisone). The period of treatment varies from patient to patient but is usually at least 6 months. The side-effects of treatment depend on the drug or drugs used and Appendix A can be used as a rough guide.

Aggressive lymphomas

Stages 1 and 2

If, after careful staging, the disease appears localized, radiotherapy is the best treatment. Two-thirds of patients with stage 1 disease and half of those with stage 2 can be cured. In some cases chemotherapy may be added to the radiation. In certain types of aggressive lymphoma additional treatment is always given and patients should discuss their treatment programme bearing in mind the exact subtype of lymphoma they have. The radiotherapy fields are similar to those used for the indolent lymphomas.

Stages 3 and 4

Many aggressive lymphomas fall into this group and combination chemotherapy (Chapter 12) is the best treatment. The chances of response to treatment depend on the particular type of lymphoma but over half of all patients will have a complete remission and nearly all patients will benefit from the treatment. Several combinations are currently being used. The drugs in the common regimes are shown below and an idea of the side-effects of the combination can be gained by looking up the individual drugs in Appendix A. The toxicity and timing (scheduling) of each combination should be discussed fully before treatment is started. Most combinations are based on the same three or four drugs, they are the most active, and all are given intermittently (usually at 3-weekly intervals) for about 6 cycles.

CHOP—Cyclophosphamide, adriamycin (hydroxydaunorubicin), vincristine (oncovin), prednisone.
C-(M)OPP—Cyclophosphamide, vincristine (oncovin), prednisone, procarbazine.
BACOP—Bleomycin, adriamycin, cyclophosphamide, vincristine (oncovin), prednisone.
COMLA—Cyclophosphamide, vincristine (oncovin), methotrexate, leucovorin, cytosine arabinoside.
CVP—Cycophosphamide, vincristine, prednisone.
M-BACOD—Methotrexate, bleomycin, adriamycin, cyclophosphamide, vincristine, DTIC.
MACOP-B—Methotrexate, adriamycin, cyclophosphamide, vincristine, prednisone, bleomycin.

Treatment is usually given for a fixed period of time and the need for further treatment then assessed. The period of treatment varies but is often six treatments, though some doctors continue treatment for 2 cycles after a complete remission (page 259) has been attained. If the particular type of lymphoma is associated with a risk of brain involvement then radiotherapy to the brain and injections by a lumbar puncture (page 201) may be given as for patients with leukaemia (page 200).

Side-effects of the chemotherapy vary from regime to regime and from person to person. The most common are:

- Tiredness and malaise—a general feeling of being unwell.
- Nausea and vomiting for some hours after each treatment.
- Loss of hair (this always happens with adriamycin, and it is also common with the other drugs).

- Risk of infection and bleeding due to low white cells and platelets (page 88).
- Tingling or weakness of the hands and feet. This takes some months to recover.

SUMMARY OF THE TREATMENT OF THE NON-HODGKIN'S LYMPHOMAS

(1) They are most common after the age of 50 years.
(2) There are many types of lymphoma which often behave in different fashions.
(3) There is no internationally accepted classification of the different types but all doctors agree on two broad types: (a) indolent lymphomas, (b) aggressive lymphomas.
(4) Treatment differs according to these two types and the spread of the disease. The same staging system is used as in Hodgkin's disease.

Indolent lymphomas

(5) Radiotherapy is used for stage 1 indolent lymphomas.
(6) Provided it is not causing symptoms or endangering the patient, more extensive indolent lymphoma (stages 2–4) can be watched initially. Treatment is reserved for progressive disease causing symptoms and can often be delayed for some years. When treatment is needed it is best to give simple treatment wherever possible. Although this type of lymphoma responds well to treatment, cure is rare.
(7) Long remissions can occur after treatment for indolent lymphomas but the disease nearly always returns.

Aggressive lymphomas

(8) Radiotherapy is used for localized (stages 1 or 2) aggressive lymphomas and may be curative in many.
(9) More extensive aggressive lymphomas should be treated with combination chemotherapy. The chance for cure depends on the particular type and amount of spread. Involvement of the lining of the brain (meninges) is relatively common with certain types of aggressive lymphoma.
(10) If a patient with an aggressive lymphoma has a relapse, it

will usually happen within one year. Those surviving without relapse for more than 2 years are probably cured.

CHAPTER 33

Acute leukaemia

Leukaemia is a cancer which develops in the bone marrow. It can roughly be divided into two main types, acute leukaemias and chronic leukaemias; this section only deals with the acute ones.

Although radiation and some drugs are known to cause acute leukaemia there is no obvious reason for the disease to develop in most patients and screening is of no use.

Most cases of acute leukaemia in adults are of a type known as acute non-lymphocytic leukaemia (also called acute myelogenous leukaemia, AML). Acute lymphocytic leukaemia, the type commonly seen in children, is seen in adults but is rare.

ACUTE NON-LYMPHOCYTIC LEUKAEMIA (ANLL OR AML)

Acute non-lymphocytic leukaemia includes acute myelogenous leukaemia, myelomonocytic leukaemia, monocytic leukaemia, promyelocytic leukaemia, and erythroleukaemia, as well as various subtypes according to the type of cell mainly involved.

SYMPTOMS

The symptoms of acute leukaemia are usually caused by a lack of normal cells in the bone marrow (page 88). About one-half of patients initially see their doctor because of a non-specific tiredness and other symptoms of anaemia. Others may develop infections (due to a lack of infection-fighting white cells) that do not respond normally to antibiotics. Some may also have bruising of the skin, bleeding from the gums or nose, or bleeding into the urine or bowel. This is caused by a lack of platelets which are blood cells needed for clotting.

DIAGNOSIS

This is usually easy to make. Any patient with symptoms suggestive of leukaemia should have a blood count. If leukaemia is present, the blood count will be abnormal with leukaemic cells (often called blasts) and reduced numbers of normal cells. If the blood count looks like leukaemia the patient should be referred to a specialist (haematologist) who will perform a bone marrow test (page 53). This is a simple, relatively painless test using a thin needle to suck marrow from a bone.

TREATMENT

Ten or more years ago there was no effective treatment for acute leukaemia and all patients died quickly. Nowadays drug treatment (chemotherapy) has greatly improved the patient's chances, though cure is rare.

Treatment is usually started soon after the diagnosis. The greatest dangers from acute leukaemia are life-threatening infections or bleeding and the patient will not improve until the disease is controlled and normal cells have returned to the blood. Because chemotherapy also reduces the number of normal cells in the blood it is common for patients to go through a prolonged period when they are very unwell and during this time they rely on the skill of their doctor to treat any infections or episodes of bleeding they may develop. Because of this need for expert support most patients are best treated in large hospitals or cancer centres.

Chemotherapy (Chapter 12)

Chemotherapy is used in several phases: induction, consolidation, and maintenance.

Induction

This is the first phase of treatment using high doses of drugs in an attempt to obtain control of the disease. This is the most risky time during treatment as many patients are already sick and the treatment increases the risk of infection or bleeding. Nearly all patients will have some of these problems.

- Excessive tiredness or weakness.
- Nausea or vomiting after treatment.
- Fevers if infected.
- Sore mouth or thrush (page 87).
- Loss of appetite.
- Loss of weight.
- Temporary loss of hair.
- Bleeding into the skin or from the gums.

Some patients die during this phase of treatment, but the alternative is nearly all the patients dying quickly if no treatment is given. Different regimes of drugs are used in different hospitals, but the most commonly used drugs are (Appendix A): daunorubicin, cytosine arabinoside, and thioguanine. One to three courses of treatment are usually needed to get the bone marrow back to normal (called a complete remission) and gaps between treatment will vary from 5 days to 14 days according to the blood count or bone marrow.

The whole of this phase is governed largely by the results of these tests so that the course of treatment cannot be predicted until their results are known. If the treatment successfully gets rid of the leukaemic cells the blood count will return to normal over the next couple of weeks. The patient will then rapidly start to feel better and the problems of infection and bleeding go away. Induction usually takes several weeks and most patients will be in hospital all or most of this time. About six to eight out of every ten patients will go into *complete remission* with induction therapy. This does not mean that they are cured, only that the doctors can see no remaining evidence of the leukaemia.

Consolidation

Because it is likely that there are a few unseen leukaemia cells left in the bone marrow, most patients receive several more treatments of high dose chemotherapy. This is known as consolidation and, despite the high doses used, it is usually much better tolerated by patients as their blood count is normal before they start treatment.

Maintenance chemotherapy

Even after consolidation therapy most patients whose bone marrow has gone back to normal (complete remission) will eventually have the disease return. In an attempt to delay this 'relapse' some doctors give their patients regular treatments of low doses of drugs. This treatment, known as maintenance therapy, is still being tested in trials and is not used by all specialists.

OUTLOOK

If treatment is not given most patients are dead within two to three months. Intensive chemotherapy produces a complete remission in 50–80 per cent of patients (this is partly dependent on age, as older patients tolerate treatment less well). Those patients who do not go into a complete remission, unfortunately, usually die quickly, often during their induction treatment. Patients in complete remission feel well and live longer (about 18 months on average) though a small proportion (less than 15 per cent) live for more than 5 years and may be cured. The majority of patients who go into complete remission will relapse, though their life may be further prolonged with chemotherapy and a second or third complete remission is not uncommon. However, the chances of improved survival must be weighed against the very unpleasant side-effects of the treatment. Unfortunately if the intensity of the treatment is reduced the chances of a remission are much less. In young patients intensive treatment is nearly always worthwhile; but the advantages and disadvantages must always be weighed carefully in older patients (more than 65 years of age) and less intensive treatment may be best.

Anyone receiving treatment for leukaemia needs a great deal of support and help from all those around them. Most feel unwell before treatment and at first are made worse by treatment. Even when the intensive first phase is over more hospital treatment, injections, and side-effects are unavoidable and emotional support is of great importance.

Bone marrow transplantation has been tested extensively in the past few years. It is only useful if a family member, who can act as a donor, has matching marrow cells. Patients are usually treated whilst in remission and it works best in patients under 35 years of age. The procedure is relatively simple, but there is always a dangerous period for at least several months after the transplant. Only a very few patients are eligible for this treatment and thorough discussion is needed before embarking on a very toxic treatment.

ACUTE LYMPHOCYTIC LEUKAEMIA (ALL)

The treatment of this type of leukaemia is similar to that of widespread aggressive lymphomas (page 192).

SYMPTOMS

These usually include:

- Enlarged lymph glands.
- Tiredness.
- Fevers and sweats.
- Bone pains.
- Symptoms from involvement of nerves, the spinal cord, or brain.
- Symptoms from an enlarged spleen.
- Symptoms from fluid or glands in the chest.

DIAGNOSIS

This is made in much the same way as non-lymphocytic leukaemia and tests include:

- Blood count.
- Bone marrow.
- Lymph node biopsy.
- Chest X-rays.
- Isotope scans or X-rays.

TREATMENT

Several drugs are used together, usually given by injection, and treatment is given about once every 3 weeks. The most commonly used drugs (Appendix A) are:

- Adriamycin.
- Cyclophosphamide.
- Vincristine.
- Methotrexate.
- Bleomycin.
- Prednisolone.

A rough idea of the side-effects of any combination of these drugs can be gained from looking up the individual drugs in Appendix A. Most patients have much less in the way of side-effects than those with acute non-lymphocytic leukaemia as the blood count is usually less abnormal when treatment starts. Despite this, treatment is intense and there are life-threatening risks from infection and bleeding.

Most patients go into a complete remission with treatment and during this period doctors usually recommend cranial prophylactic radiotherapy and chemotherapy (page 252) to try to prevent spread to the brain. Radiotherapy takes about 2 weeks and causes little toxicity.

Maintenance therapy is also used by some doctors in this type of leukaemia. Patients relapsing from a complete remission can be put into a further remission with more chemotherapy though it is likely to last for a progressively shorter time with each relapse. The leukaemia may also spread to the nervous system and this may become a difficult problem to treat. Injections of drugs (intrathecal injection—page 252) into the fluid around the brain and spinal cord are used often with radiotherapy. Unfortunately they are usually only of temporary benefit and the disease eventually returns in the nervous system or blood.

The chances of cure for acute lymphocytic leukaemia in adults is very much less than in children (page 250) and it is a much more resistant disease. However, more encouraging results have recently been reported in some hospitals and the treatment continues to improve.

SUMMARY OF THE TREATMENT OF ACUTE LEUKAEMIA IN ADULTS

(1) There are two major types: (a) the common acute non-lymphocytic leukaemia and (b) the rare acute lymphocytic leukaemia.

Acute non-lymphocytic leukaemia

(2) Some chemicals and irradiation can cause this leukaemia.

(3) Screening is not helpful.

(4) Patients are often very ill before treatment starts and most will die quickly without therapy.

(5) Intensive chemotherapy is used to treat the disease and this often makes patients more unwell and some die during this stage of treatment.

(6) Between 60 to 80 per cent of younger patients will obtain a complete remission. They feel well during this time though remission is usually temporary. A small number of patients have long remission (more than 5 years).

(7) After relapse some patients can obtain a further remission.

(8) The severe side-effects of the treatment must be weighed against the potential benefits—especially in the elderly.

Acute lymphocytic leukaemia in adults

(9) This is a much more resistant disease than in children.

(10) It is treated with combinations of several drugs.

(11) Side-effects are usually less than in acute non-lymphocytic leukaemia.

(12) There is a risk of central nervous system involvement and cranial radiation and intrathecal drugs are often given to try to prevent this.

(13) Most patients go into a complete remission though this is usually temporary.

CHAPTER 34

Chronic leukaemia

Chronic leukaemias can broadly be divided into two main types according to the type of blood cell involved: (a) myelocytes—chronic myloid leukaemia, (b) lymphocytes—chronic lymphatic leukaemia. Because their treatment and course is different they will be discussed separately.

CHRONIC MYELOID LEUKAEMIA (CML)

Another name for this condition is chronic granulocytic leukaemia (CGL) and the terms are interchangeable. It is most common in middle age but can occur at any age. No cause is known and screening is not helpful.

SYMPTOMS

These are often just a vague feeling of malaise and include:

- Tiredness.
- Shortness of breath.
- Weight loss.
- Loss of appetite.
- Fevers and sweats.
- Pain in the left side of the abdomen from an enlarged spleen.
- Occasionally nose bleeds or bruising.

DIAGNOSIS

This is usually fairly easy. A blood count will show increased numbers of neutrophils (infection-fighting white cells) and sometimes anaemia or a reduction in the number of platelets (clotting cells). Because this picture may be similar to that seen in the blood during an infection, a bone marrow test (page 53) is needed to be certain of the diagnosis. Special chemical tests (leucocyte alkaline phosphatase) are used to help make the diagnosis and the chromosomes (carrying the genetic code) are examined. Nearly all patients with this type of leukaemia have a special abnormality of their chromosomes called a Philadelphia chromosome.

TREATMENT

Because many patients with this type of chronic leukaemia feel unwell they are usually given drug treatment. Unfortunately it is not possible to eradicate the leukaemia from the bone marrow and to cure patients. Treatment can, however, control the disease and get rid of symptoms and return people to a normal life.

Chemotherapy (Chapter 12)

As the treatment is palliative (to get rid of symptoms) a simple oral treatment is usually used. The most widely used drug is busulphan (Appendix A). This is available in tablets of differing strength and it is given to patients until the white blood count falls to nearly normal levels. A reduced dose is then commonly used to try to keep the blood count near normal. It is important to have regular blood tests while on treatment so that the correct dose can be given. The tablets are usually remarkably well tolerated and disease may be controlled for long periods. Other drugs can also be used with good results.

Surgery (Chapter 10)

Because the spleen of patients with CML can become painfully enlarged it is sometimes removed surgically. This can be very helpful in selected patients.

Radiotherapy (Chapter 11)

Radiotherapy may be used to treat a painful enlarged spleen. As well as shrinking the spleen, it also reduces the white blood count and improves the bone marrow.

OUTLOOK

Although it is a chronic disease that is well controlled by simple therapy many patients eventually develop a more aggressive type of leukaemia (accelerated phase). This is usually very difficult to control even when it is treated in the same way as acute myelogenous leukaemia. Despite this, about one in five patients in this 'accelerated phase' respond well to treatment. These patients can usually be picked out on blood and bone marrow tests as their abnormal cells look more like lymphocytes.

The outlook is therefore variable. Control of the disease and symptomatic improvement for a number of years is achieved in most patients but an aggressive and usually untreatable acute leukaemia eventually develops in most patients. Bone marrow transplanation has been used in selected patients with some encouraging results.

CHRONIC LYMPHCYTIC LEUKAEMIA

This is a disease which produces less symptoms and in a good proportion of patients the disease is only found when a routine blood test turns out to be abnormal. It is most common in the elderly but can occur at any age.

SYMPTOMS

These are variable but most patients only have relatively mild problems which may include:

- Generalized tiredness.
- Swollen lymph glands which are usually painless.
- Fevers and sweats.
- Uncommonly anaemia, bruising, or bleeding.
- Recurrent infections.

DIAGNOSIS

This is usually simple as a blood count will show increased numbers of lymphocytes (a type of white cell). However, a bone marrow test (page 53) is needed to be sure of the diagnosis and sometimes a lymph node biopsy is done.

TREATMENT

This is an indolent disease that often requires no therapy for long periods. Because the aim of therapy is to control symptoms treatment is usually not given until a problem develops. This may include:

- Large lymph nodes pressing on an important part of the body (e.g. obstruction of a ureter, the tube from kidney to bladder).
- Debilitating symptoms such as weight loss, fevers, and sweats.
- Anaemia or low platelets.
- Serious recurrent infections.

Cure is unfortunately not possible, but good control of symptoms can be expected.

Chemotherapy (Chapter 12)

The most commonly used drugs are chlorambucil and the steroid prednisone, though any alkylating agent (Appendix A) can be used instead of chlorambucil. The treatment is usually given orally in low doses though high dose intermittent treatment may occasionally be given if a rapid response is required.

Radiotherapy (Chapter 11)

This is rarely used as primary treatment but radiation to bulky troublesome nodes can be helpful in some cases.

This type of chronic leukaemia, unlike chronic granulocytic leukaemia, does not usually change into an acute form. However, it may with time become increasingly dificult to treat because the bone marrow is unable to work properly. This results in anaemia, a tendency of bleeding (low platelets), and a tendency to infection. These all make it dificult to give chemotherapy as such treatment will make these problems worse, certainly in the short run.

OUTLOOK

This is a chronic disease and most patients will survive for five or more years even with no treatment.

CHAPTER 35

Multiple myeloma

This is a cancer of the plasma cells in the bone marrow which is most common between the ages of 50 and 65 years. Plasma cells develop from lymphocytes and produce antibodies which fight infections. Because patients cannot make normal antibodies they are very susceptible to infections. The cause of myeloma is not known and screening is of no help.

SYMPTOMS

The disease usually involves bones all over the body though it may very occasionally be confined to one part of the body. The common symptoms are:

- Pain or discomfort in a bone.
- Recurrent infections that do not respond normally to antibiotics.
- Bones that break (fracture) after little or no injury.
- Shortness of breath.
- Undue tiredness.

DIAGNOSIS

This may be suspected on a routine blood count but special tests are needed to confine the diagnosis. These include:

- Bone marrow (page 53) to look at the plasma cells.
- Blood test to examine blood proteins (plasma electrophoresis).
- X-rays of bones and sometimes a bone scan (page 49).

TREATMENT

Because the bone marrow is usually extensively involved drug treatment is needed. Even though discomfort is a problem it is best to avoid staying in bed as this may make things worse as the blood calcium may rise (page 274).

Chemotherapy (Chapter 12)

The majority of patients will respond to simple treatment with tablets. The most commonly used drugs are melphalan (Appendix A) and the steroid prednisolone. They are usually given once every 4 to 6 weeks. Occasionally several drugs given by injection may be used if the disease does not respond to melphalan treatment.

Most patients feel better and live longer because of treatment. This response often lasts several years.

Radiation (Chapter 11)

Radiotherapy is very effective treatment for a pain confined to a bone. Most patients respond quickly and short courses of treatment will produce dramatic results with almost no side-effects.

OUTLOOK

Although myeloma responds to simple treatment it unfortunately usually escapes control after a variable period (years in most cases). It is then difficult to treat and the aim should be designed to control specific symptoms.

The problems associated with uncontrolled disease are:

- Bone pain—usually well controlled by radiotherapy.
- Recurrent infections.
- Anaemia.
- Bruising or bleeding (low platelets).
- Generalized tiredness and weakness.
- Raised calcium in the blood.

CHAPTER 36

Rodent ulcers and squamous cancer of the skin

Both of these tumours grow slowly and only spread to other parts of the body late in their course. They remain localized for long periods but if they are neglected they will become incurable. Delayed treatment also means that more normal tissue must be removed with the cancer and this may be disfiguring, especially if it involves the face.

SYMPTOMS

A basal cell cancer usually develops in an area of skin exposed to sunlight and begins as a small firm protuberance that may ulcerate in the middle as it grows. The edges of the lump are often raised and it is said to look waxy or pearly.

Squamous cell cancers also grow on sun-exposed areas. They often develop in pre-cancerous skin lesions called solar (sun) or senile keratoses. At first it appears as a hard scaly lesion that as it enlarges breaks down in the centre and ulcerates and becomes covered by a scab. Only if the diagnosis of cancer is long delayed is tumour spread likely.

DIAGNOSIS

Anybody with a skin lesion that enlarges or ulcerates should go to their doctor, though many of these do not turn out to be cancer. If it is cancer the chances of cure are good but are much better if there is no delay in diagnosis. Any suspicious lump should be biopsied and usually no further investigations are needed unless the lump is large or there is evidence of spread to nearby lymph nodes.

TREATMENT

The aim of treatment is removal of all the cancer with a margin of normal tissue. The way this is done will depend on where the cancer is and how large it is. The following techniques are available.

Excisional surgery (Chapter 10)

This is simply cutting out the lump. If the cancer is small the edges of the wound can be stitched together, but if it is large a skin graft is often needed. Most operations of this type can be done under a local anaesthetic.

Electrosurgery

This is the use of an electric needle that burns away the cancer. This is only used for small tumours and several treatments are often necessary. However, it can be done under a local anaesthetic and can be very useful in selected cases.

Cryosurgery

This is the use of liquid nitrogen to kill the cancer by freezing. It is usually reserved for pre-malignant lesions and very small cancers.

Radiotherapy (Chapter 11)

Radiation can be used to treat skin cancers but because treatment takes 3–4 weeks it is more troublesome. However, in certain situations such as tumours of the face it may avoid disfiguring surgery.

A tumour that has spread is more dificult to cure. It usually spreads to the lymph nodes and an operation to remove the cancer and its draining lymph nodes may be done, an 'en bloc resection'. Radiotherapy may be of some use but chemotherapy is ineffective and toxic treatment should be avoided.

If a tumour is detected early the chance of cure is over 90 per cent; but if the local lymph nodes are affected the cure rate falls to 50 per cent. Skin cancer that has spread to other parts of the body is rarely cured.

SUMMARY OF THE TREATMENT OF SKIN CANCER

See the summary at the end of Chapter 37 (page 215).

Malignant melanoma

Fortunately, this type of skin cancer is less common as it is much more malignant. It usually occurs in areas exposed to the sun but can grow anywhere. The tumour develops in the pigmented cells in the skin and many start in moles or birthmarks. Although most people have moles the chances of one becoming cancerous are small and the routine removal of moles is not justified.

SYMPTOMS

Any mole that develops or changes must be examined by a doctor. Any of the following symptoms may be important.

- Irritation.
- Itching.
- Soreness.
- Change in size.
- Change in colour (darker or lighter).
- Bleeding.
- New moles around it.

Malignant melanomas often spread quickly and the key to cure is early diagnosis. Any suspicious moles or pigmented lesions must be examined.

DIAGNOSIS AND TREATMENT

If a malignant melanoma is suspected the patient should be referred to a dermatologist or a surgeon. The suspected lesion should be completely removed and then examined under a microscope. Some surgeons may take a small margin of tissue with the mole but if it is shown to be a malignant melanoma they will need to do a further operation to remove a wide margin of normal tissue. Other surgeons, if they think it is malignant will take a wide margin of tissue at the first operation. In Australia special clinics have been set up to try to detect early cases. Anyone who is worried about a skin change can go to these clinics and this, together with an increased public awareness of skin cancer, has improved the cure rate for melanoma.

Surgery (Chapter 10)

A good operation must include the removal of the melanoma with a 2–4 cm margin of tissue around it and the resulting wound usually needs a skin graft to help healing. The chances of cure depend very much on how deeply the cancer has penetrated the skin.

There is still argument amongst surgeons about whether it is a good thing to remove the nearby lymph nodes (page 23). This is only useful if the mole develops on a leg or arm as in other parts of the body the tumour can spread to different groups of lymph nodes. There are no definite guidelines for when a lymph node resection should be done, but if it is planned the operation should only be done by an experienced cancer surgeon.

Radiotherapy (Chapter 11)

On the whole these cancers are not very responsive to radiation. However, if large fractions (big doses at each treatment) are given tumours can be controlled. Radiotherapy is usually reserved for selected malignant melanomas of the face (where surgery would be disfiguring) and to treat some recurrent tumours. Repeated treatments are required over a couple of weeks but only about ten fractions are needed as the dose of each fraction is higher than usual.

Chemotherapy (Chapter 12)

Unfortunately drug treatment for this cancer is not good. Several drugs can shrink tumours in about one in five patients but combinations of the drugs do not improve on this and, on the whole, toxic treatment should be avoided. The side-effects of the commonly used drugs can be found in Appendix A.

Immunotherapy

This is the use of various treatments to improve the immune system's ability to naturally destroy the tumour. Though some types of immunotherapy can shrink the tumour if it is used directly on the cancer there is no good evidence that the chance of cure is improved.

The chances of cure for malignant melanoma are dependent on:

- Early diagnosis.
- The depth of penetration through the skin of the cancer.
- Good surgery.

Cure is unlikely if the cancer is shown to have spread. The tests that may be used to detect spread include:

- Chest X-ray.
- Liver ultrasound (page 45) or isotope scan (page 50).
- Bone scan (page 49).
- CT Brain scan (page 47).

However, malignant melanoma is a strange cancer and widespread disease can, rarely, undergo spontaneous regression for years. Conversely other patients, apparently cured years ago, may have a tumour which suddenly recurs.

SUMMARY OF THE TREATMENT OF SKIN CANCER

(1) Fair-skinned people are more prone to develop skin cancer if their skin is exposed to sunlight.
(2) Any non-healing skin lesion or changing mole should be examined by a doctor—preferably a dermatologist.
(3) Basal cell and squamous skin cancers are just about the most curable of all tumours, but if diagnosis is delayed they can kill. Most patients are cured by a simple procedure to remove the cancer.
(4) Malignant melanoma develops in pigment cells and spreads rapidly.
(5) A wide excision of the melanoma is needed and this often means a skin graft. A specialist surgeon is often required.

(6) Radiotherapy is not usually used for treatment but can be helpful for recurrent lesions.

(7) Chemotherapy is not very useful and toxic treatment should be avoided.

(8) Immunotherapy remains unproven.

(9) The course of widespread melanoma is unpredictable.

CHAPTER 38

Brain

Brain tumours are very frightening, but many are not malignant. Those that are, may arise within the brain itself (a primary brain tumour) or grow elsewhere and then spread to the brain (a secondary brain tumour). Cancers of the lung, breast, and malignant melanomas as well as lymphomas and leukemias are the tumours most prone to spread to the brain. Primary brain tumours, in contrast, rarely spread beyond the central nervous system (the brain and spinal cord).

The brain and spinal cord is surrounded by a protective bony case, the skull and spine. Neither of these allows much room for expansion so that tumours of the central nervous system quickly cause pressure symptoms as they expand.

PRIMARY BRAIN TUMOURS

The chance of cure depends on the type of tumour and where it is in the brain. Tumours on the surface of the brain are easier to operate on, whilst it is often too dangerous to remove deep tumours. This is because many deep structures in the brain are essential for life and cannot be operated on. Benign tumours are usually on the surface of the brain (the commonest is called a meningioma) but unfortunately many cancers are deep in the brain and invade surrounding tissue.

Symptoms

Brain tumours cause symptoms either by invading the tissues in the area of the brain in which it is growing or by the increased pressure it causes within the skull. The symptoms caused by the local growth of tumour vary according to which part of the brain is affected. Because of this symptoms are very varied and it is not possible to list the possible effects. One specific problem may, however, be seizures or epileptic fits. Seizures are caused by an area of irritation in the brain though it is worth remembering that most epileptics do not have cancer. Despite this all adults who develop epilepsy should have tests to rule out a tumour. The major symptoms caused by increased pressure within the skull (called raised intracranial pressure) are headache, nausea and vomiting, and slowly increasing mental confusion.

Headaches

Everyone gets a headache from time to time and only very, very rarely is this due to a tumour; so it can usually be ignored. Severe persistent or increasing headaches should, however, be investigated but remember that there are *many* causes of which a brain tumour is only one.

Diagnosis

When a brain tumour is suspected, a neurologist, who is a doctor specializing in the care and diagnosis of diseases of the central nervous system, will be asked to see the patient. If, after talking to and examining a patient he feels there is a significant abnormality these tests may be arranged.

- X-ray of the skull. Some tumours may show up as they contain calcium (like bones) and others, although not visible, may push the structures of the brain to one side. Signs of increased pressure may also be seen.
- Electroencephalogram (EEG). This is a recording of the brain waves or electrical activity of the brain. During the test, wires are tapped to various parts of the skull and may show an abnormal pattern if there is a cancer. The test is simple and entirely safe, but is less useful now new X-ray techniques are available.
- Brain scan (page 52). Brain tumours have a rich blood supply and the radioactivity that is injected acumulates in the cancer and shows up as an area of increased radioactivity (a hot spot).
- CT scan (page 47). This gives a very detailed picture of the brain and can detect a small tumour and the excess fluid (oedema) that usually surrounds it. An injection of contrast

dye may be given into an arm vein to highlight the cancer. This causes a short-lived sensation of being hot all over.

- Arteriogram (page 41). If a tumour has shown up an X-ray to outline the blood vessels within the tumour may be done. This not only shows up the exact location of the tumour but also reveals the blood vessels supplying it. This may be useful to a neurosurgeon planning an operation. The technique of the test will depend on which artery is to be examined and it is worth discussing the test before admission to hospital.

- Tests to exclude a secondary tumour. Before deciding if an operation is advisable the neurosurgeon will consider whether the tumour is primary or secondary. Patients should be asked if they have had any other cancer and will be examined with particular attention being paid to the lungs (chest X-ray), skin (looking for malignant melanoma) and the breasts; urine will also be checked for any blood in case there is a kidney tumour. If these tests are normal it is unlikely that the tumour has spread to the brain.

Treatment

This depends on the type of tumour and should always be done in a neurosurgical centre or a children's cancer centre.

Gliomas

These are the commonest brain tumours and are most often seen between the ages of 30 and 60 years, though they are also common in children. Important factors affecting the chances of cure are:

- Site of the tumour. Some are easily removed but, unfortunately, most are deep in the brain and cannot be completely excised.

- The appearance under a microscope. Some tumours do not look very abnormal (grade 1) whilst others may be very malignant-looking (grade 4). Usually the higher the grade (1–4), the faster-growing is the tumour and the worse the outlook.

The first treatment is medical. A steroid drug, dexamethasone is given by mouth to reduce any swelling in the brain. It does not shrink the tumour but decreases the fluid (oedema) around it. If the patient has had seizures (fits), antiepileptic drugs (phenobarbitone and/or phenytoin) are given to prevent more.

Surgery (Chapter 12)

Surgery will be considered. Most tumours cannot be cured this way, but some can if all the cancer is removed. It is not possible to describe such operations in detail, but an attempt to remove all or as much as possible of the tumour is often made. Before such an operation the hair must be shaved off (it will grow back normally afterwards) and then under an anaesthetic a flap of scalp is lifted up and a small section of the skull over the tumour is removed. The tumour and surrounding normal brain tissue is then removed and the piece of skull is then replaced and the scalp is stitched up.

One of the potential problems of brain surgery is the possibility of further neurological damage caused by removing normal brain tissue with the tumour. The likelihood of damage depends on where the tumour is and with some tumours the risk may be very small. There is often further swelling of the brain for a few days after an operation and this can cause symptoms to temporarily get worse. As well as the usual improvement due to the swelling getting better, the brain can often adjust to damage and, with intensive rehabilitation, the symptoms of local brain damage may recover.

Chemotherapy (Chapter 12)

Drug treatment remains experimental. Few drugs are active in these tumours, the most commonly used ones are BCNU and CCNU (Appendix A). Their effects are modest but they do cause nausea and vomiting together with bone marrow damage so that the advantages and disadvantages of treatment must be discussed before it is started.

Outlook

Some patients with low grade tumours are cured whilst the others can live for years. If the tumour is of higher grade then the outlook is, unfortunately, poorer with few patients surviving two years, though occasional patients can be cured if the tumour can be completely removed.

Medulloblastoma

This is a tumour of young children which usually grows in the part of the brain concerned with coordination (the cerebellum) and because of this, a common symptom is incoordination. They are fast growing and unlike other brain tumours spread to other parts of the brain and spinal cord. Despite its high degree of malignancy it is possible to cure this tumour.

Treatment should always be in a specialist centre and includes a combination of surgery, radiotherapy, and often chemotherapy. Surgery confirms the diagnosis and as much tumour as possible is removed. After surgery, radiotherapy is given both to the brain and to the whole of the spine. High doses of radiotherapy are given to the main tumour and this takes about 6 to 8 weeks. Lower doses are given to the rest of the central nervous system over 4 to 5 weeks. Chemotherapy drugs (Chapter 12) are usually given into a vein or into the fluid around the spinal cord (an intrathecal injection into the CSF). It is obvious that the treatment of this type of brain tumour is highly complex and children should always go to a special cancer centre for treatment. Not only do they need expertise in arranging the best treatment, they and their family will also require special rehabilitation and support that is usually only available in such a centre.

One of the long-term effects of radiotherapy (Chapter 11) is slowing normal bone growth. Because of this children who have radiotherapy to their spine as infants tend to be short and can develop curvature of the spine if care is not taken. Despite the complexity of the treatment and its side-effects, over half of these children are alive after five years and more and more children are being cured. Parents must discuss all aspects of the treatment for this cancer before it is started as it requires a great commitment from everyone involved.

SECONDARY TUMOURS OF THE BRAIN

Spread of a tumour to the brain is even more common than a tumour developing in the brain itself. The symptoms are similar to those of a primary brain tumour but in addition there may be effects from the primary tumour. Occasionally the first signs of cancer are symptoms caused by secondary spread to the brain, but in most cases the patient is already known to have a cancer. Investigations include:

- Skull X-ray.
- CT scan (page 47) or brain scan (page 52).
- Possibly an arteriogram (page 41) if surgery is contemplated.
- Investigation of the primary tumour.

Treatment depends very much on what is happening to the primary cancer, but usually radiotherapy is given and this will control symptoms for a time. When the main tumour is uncontrolled the aim of treatment is to improve symptoms. If the patient is *entirely* free of other cancer and there is only a solitary brain secondary an operation may be attempted. If patients are selected carefully such an operation can be very useful, some patients living for extra years whilst some may be cured. However, surgical removal of a secondary brain tumour is very much the exception rather than the rule.

OTHER MALIGNANT TUMOURS OF THE BRAIN

There are a number of uncommon primary brain tumours but space does not allow discussion of their treatment. They include:

(1) Teratomas.
(2) Pineliomas.
(3) Neurolemmaomas and other rare tumours.

BENIGN TUMOURS OF THE BRAIN

Benign tumours do not grow or behave like cancer but because they cause pressure within the skull they do need urgent treatment. They can usually be treated successfully by surgery or radiotherapy and never spread. The common tumours falling into this group include:

(1) Meningiomas (tumours of the lining over the brain).

(2) Pituitary tumours (the pituitary is a small gland at the base of the brain that controls the other glands in the body).

(3) Acoustic neuroma (a benign tumour of the nerve from the ear to the brain).

SUMMARY OF THE TREATMENT OF BRAIN TUMOURS

(1) Brain tumours may arise in the brain itself (primary) or spread from another cancer (secondary).

(2) The skull and spine enclose the brain and spinal cord so that a tumour quickly causes symptoms of increased pressure.

(3) Symptoms are caused by the local effects of the tumour (this includes seizures) and by the raised pressure.

(4) The commonest primary tumours are gliomas. They are usually not curable though superficial low grade tumours can be cured by complete surgical removal. People with low grade tumours may live for years after partial surgical removal and radiotherapy but high grade tumours are usually rapidly fatal.

(5) Chemotherapy may be helpful to a few patients. More important drugs are dexamethasone (to reduce oedema) and antiepileptics to control seizures if they occur.

(6) Medulloblastoma is a very malignant brain tumour of children. Treatment, which is complex, including surgery, radiotherapy, and chemotherapy and should be given in a children's cancer centre. Despite its rapid growth and tendency to spread, it is curable.

(7) Spread of cancer to the brain is more common than are primary brain tumours and treatment is influenced by the state of the primary tumour. Usually radiotherapy is used to control symptoms but occasionally an operation to completely remove a single brain metastasis may cure a patient if the primary tumour is controlled.

(8) *Benign* tumours rapidly cause symptoms and should be treated as quickly as possible. Surgery or radiotherapy can cure or control the disease for many years.

CHAPTER 39

Thyroid

The thyroid gland lies in the neck just below the larynx (voice box) and produces a hormone which regulates the body's rate of metabolism. Swellings of the thyroid are common and most are not due to cancer. If you have a lump in your thyroid consult your doctor to find out what it is, but do not be too concerned about cancer as thyroid tumours are rare.

The only known cause of thyroid cancer is exposure to radiation. In the past, it was popular to irradiate the thymus (a gland in the chest) of children will all sorts of illnesses and it seems that these children are more likely to develop thyroid cancer.

SYMPTOMS

Many thyroid cancers are found because of swelling of the neck. There are different types of thyroid swelling; if it is diffuse throughout the gland it is unlikely to be a cancer. If one part of the gland is enlarged, it is called a nodule. This may be benign or malignant and may or may not produce thyroid hormone. If it does produce hormone this causes hyper-thyroidism (over-active thyroid) the symptoms of which are:

- Nervousness.
- Intolerance of warm weather.
- Weight loss.
- Weakness.
- Rapid pulse or palpitations.
- Diarrhoea.

If the thyroid nodule produces hormone it is very unlikely to be malignant. Non-hormone producing nodules may be a simple cyst or may be cancer. Rare symptoms of advanced thyroid cancer include hoarseness.

DIAGNOSIS

This is made by a combination of physical examination and a thyroid scan (page 51). A scan will show up an over-active nodule as a hot spot and a non-functioning one as a cold spot. An ultrasound examination (page 45) may be done to see if a non-functioning nodule is a cyst or not. If a thyroid cancer is found it may be described, after examination under a microscope, as papillary (least malignant), follicular, or anaplastic (most malignant).

TREATMENT

Surgery (Chapter 10)

Thyroid cancer that remains localized to the gland itself can be cured by an operation to remove the thyroid (a thyroidectomy). The extent of the operation remains debatable and while some surgeons may leave some of the gland behind (a partial thyroidectomy) others will remove all of the gland and the neighbouring glands (a total thyroidectomy and excision of lymph nodes).

Potential problems of thyroid surgery include:

(1) Decrease or lack of thyroid hormone, leading to hypothyroidism (symptoms: slowness, intolerance of cold, thickening of skin, loss of hair, and constipation). Replacement thyroid tablets are needed for life and allow an entirely normal life style.
(2) Changes in balance of the body's calcium salts. Small glands, called parathyroid glands located in the thyroid may be inadvertently taken out or damaged during the operation. If they are removed the blood calcium falls (hypoparathyroidism) and this can cause muscular twitching, weakness, and seizures. Supplements of vitamin D and calcium will usually control the symptoms.
(3) Damage to the nerves to the larynx (voice box) may lead to permanent hoarseness.

Most patients, happily, do not suffer serious problems after thyroidectomy and for many it offers a high chance of cure. In patients with anaplastic cancers the tumour has nearly always spread early and an operation is not helpful.

Radiation therapy (Chapter 11)

This is usually not used in the initial treatment of thyroid cancer but may be helpful in locally controlling anaplastic cancers.

Treatment of thyroid cancer that has spread (metastatic cancer)

Papillary and follicular cancers may take up iodine like a normal gland (this can be seen on an isotope scan—page 51) and because of this they can be treated with radioactive iodine. In order to treat metastatic tumour, a low dose of radioactive iodine is used to destroy the normal thyroid. No thyroid replacement is given and a high dose of radioactive iodine is then given monthly until the tumour no longer absorbs it. This is checked by repeated scans.

The radioactive iodine gives a localized but very high dose of radiation to the cancer. Although it rarely cures, it can control the tumour for years; patients will need replacement thyroid hormone tablets for life.

Occasionally the growth of thyroid cancers is partly controlled by a hormone called thyroid stimulating hormone. Levels of this hormone can be reduced by giving high doses of thyroid hormone and this may cause some tumours to shrink.

Chemotherapy (drug treatment—Chapter 12) is not very useful and only helps about one in five patients. The most commonly used drug is adriamycin (Appendix A) but toxic chemotherapy should be avoided.

OUTLOOK WITH THYROID CANCER

This is often a slow-growing cancer and the chances of cure with surgery are good. Widespread disease can frequently be controlled for years, though the outlook for those with an anaplastic cancer is unfortunately much worse.

SUMMARY OF THE TREATMENT OF THYROID CANCER

(1) Thyroid lumps are very common; very few are cancerous.
(2) Radiation of the neck may cause thyroid cancer many years later.

(3) Most cancers of the thyroid do not produce hormone.
(4) A thyroid scan will often show up the tumour.
(5) If the cancer is confined to the thyroid, removal of the gland gives a good chance of cure.
(6) Radiotherapy may be helpful in anaplastic cancers that spread rapidly.
(7) Radioactive iodine may be used to treat tumours that will absorb the iodine.
(8) Drug therapy is rarely helpful.
(9) The chance of cure is best if the cancer has not spread outside the gland.

CHAPTER 40

Cancer in children

The next eight chapters (Chapter 41 to 48) discuss the most common cancers that affect children. Fortunately cancer in children is rare and this is the group of tumours where the most progress has been made and the chances of cure are highest. Treatment is best carried out at a specialist centre where staff are experienced in dealing with the complex treatments and can give the necessary emotional support to the whole family. Table 5 lists the commonest childhood cancers. When special tests are needed in young children they will usually be done with a general anaesthetic.

| Table 5 Relative frequency (per cent) of the common childhood cancers ||
Tumour type	Relative proportion (%)
Leukaemia	30
Lymphoma	8
Hodgkin's disease	6
Nervous system tumours	12
Bone sarcoma	12
Soft tissue sarcoma	12
Neuroblastoma	10
Wilm's(kidney)	8
Others	2

CHAPTER 41

Neuroblastoma

About one in ten cases of childhood cancer is a neuroblastoma. The tumour grows from cells that form special nerves called sympathetic nerves. Because these tissues are widespread the tumour can arise in many sites, but most are at the back of the abdomen and nearly half are in an adrenal gland just above a kidney.

The cancer tends to spread locally by lymphatics (page 23) and by the blood so that it may already affect different parts of the body at diagnosis. It is most common very early in life and half of all patients are younger than 2 years of age; fortunately the outlook is best in these very young children.

This tumour often produces substances (called cate-cholamines) that may be measured in the urine. They can be helpful in establishing the diagnosis and following its response to treatment. They may also cause an increase in blood pressure as they are similar to adrenalin. It should always be remembered that very young children (less than 1 year) have a very good chance of cure even if the tumour is widespread.

SYMPTOMS

These may be caused by the local tumour or may be due to spread of the cancer. The commonest effects are:

- Swelling of the abdomen or a lump in the abdomen.
- Swelling in the neck.
- Prolonged jaundice after birth.
- Cough, shortness of breath.
- High blood pressure.
- Weight loss.
- Poor appetite.
- Protrusion of an eye (exophthalmos) caused by a tumour behind the eye.

DIAGNOSIS AND STAGING

The aim of investigation is to confirm the diagnosis and then to see if there is any spread of the cancer. A biopsy is needed before treatment is finally planned but in many cases the diagnosis will be suspected strongly before this is done.

Routine investigations include some of the following tests:

- X-ray of chest and abdomen. About half of the tumours contain some calcium (like bone) which shows up on a plain X-ray. X-rays of bone may also show spread of the tumour.
- IVP (page 34). This often shows that the kidney is pushed over by the tumour.
- 24 hours urine collection. About 8 in 10 patients will have extra amounts of catecholamines (one of which is called VMA) in their urine and this can be measured. Before such a urine test it is important that the child is on a special diet. The following foods should **not** be eaten as they will affect the test, which is often called a VMA test.

(1) Tea.
(2) Coca Cola and other colas.
(3) Chocolate.
(4) Vanilla.
(5) Bananas.
(6) Grapes.
(7) Oranges.
(8) Tomatoes.
(9) Aspirin.
(10) Sulphur antibiotics.
(11) Some cough mixtures.

- Arteriography (page 41). An arteriogram outlining the blood supply of the tumour is often useful. A general anaesthetic will usually be given.
- Lymphangiography (page 38) may be used to outline lymph nodes in the abdomen and is usually done under a general anaesthetic. Alternatively a CT scan (page 47) may be used.
- Bone marrow aspirate (page 53). This is done under a general anaesthetic and may show spread to the bone marrow.

TREATMENT

Surgery (Chapter 10)

It a child does not have any spread of the tumour and the tumour can be totally removed the cure rate is about 90 per cent, regardless of age. However, if only part of the tumour can be removed it is better only to do a biopsy to confirm the diagnosis. Operations to remove part of this tumour are usually not helpful; following biopsy metal clips will be used to mark out the area of the cancer. These will show up on an X-ray and help with radiotherapy planning. Sometimes another operation may be considered after radiotherapy and chemotherapy.

The nature of any operation depends on the size and site of the tumour but young children are very resilient and are able to stand up to major operations.

Radiotherapy (Chapter 11)

Radiotherapy may be used to treat any tumour left behind after an incomplete operation or a tumour which could not be removed at all. The radiotherapy may be given with the intention of cure or for palliation (treatment of symptoms); this depends on the size of the cancer and where it is. If a surgeon has marked out the tumour with metal clips this helps in the treatment planning.

The tumour is usually quite sensitive to irradiation and low doses may be given; older children tend to have less sensitive tumours which need more irradiation.

The treatment is usually given over 3 to 4 weeks in small divided doses. Details of the treatment programme should be discussed fully before treatment as it needs to be tailored for the individual patient. Radiotherapy is usually well tolerated but needs care in planning as it can damage bone growth.

Chemotherapy (Chapter 12)

Drug therapy is usually given in a treatment programme including surgery and radiotherapy. Although tumours often respond to treatment the chances of a complete remission (page 259) and cure are not good if the tumour is very extensive.

Various combinations of drugs are used and an idea of the side-effects of a combination can be gathered by looking up the individual drugs in Appendix A. Although chemotherapy has many side-effects, young children usually cope with these better than adults.

CHANCES OF CURE

The chance of cure depends on several factors.

(1) Age. The younger a child is the greater are the chances of survival. For those children less than 1 year about eight of every ten are cured. After this age the chance of cure gradually diminishes.
(2) Stage. The degree of spread of neuroblastoma is broken down into four stages and the higher the stage the less is the chance for cure.

In the group of very young children (less than 1 year) spontaneous regressions are quite common. A special stage (IV–S) is used to pick out young children who have widespread disease and who are likely to be cured with minimal treatment.

SUMMARY OF THE TREATMENT OF NEUROBLASTOMAS

(1) Most occur in the abdomen, usually around the adrenal gland, though they can grow in the chest or head and neck.
(2) Many of these tumours produce substances (catecholamines) that can be found in the urine. These can be used to help make the diagnosis and to follow the progress of the child.
(3) Surgery is used to make the diagnosis (biopsy) and if possible to completely remove the cancer.
(4) Radiotherapy is given for tumours that cannot be surgically taken away.
(5) Drug therapy is not very active but is often used together with surgery and radiotherapy.
(6) Despite the intensive treatment most children are able to tolerate it as they are more resilient than adults.

(7) The chance for cure is best in very young patients.

(8) A special stage (IVS) is used to describe the widespread disease in infants less than 1 year that may go away by itself (a spontaneous regression) and therefore needs little treatment.

(9) This cancer should be treated in a special centre.

(10) The whole family needs the support of their own doctor and the team treating the child.

CHAPTER 42

Wilm's tumour

Wilm's tumour, also known as nephroblastoma, is one of the commonest cancers in children usually occurring between the ages of one to five years. Although *most* children do not have any obvious genetic abnormality, Wilm's tumour is more common in children with the following unusual birth abnormalities:

(1) Abnormalities of the urogenital system (kidney, ureters, and bladder).
(2) Over-growth one half of the body (hemihypertrophy).
(3) Partial or complete absence of the iris in the eye.

SYMPTOMS

This cancer can cause several non-specific symptoms. These include abdominal discomfort, gastrointestinal upset, fever, and blood in the urine (haematuria). However, accidental discovery of a lump in the abdomen is often the first sign of the tumour. It is usually felt as a firm, irregular, and non-tender mass. In some children both kidneys may be affected.

DIAGNOSIS

If a Wilm's tumour is suspected a series of X-rays and scans (under general anaesthetic, if required) are used to try to confirm the diagnosis before any operation is contemplated. X-rays will include the following:

- A plain X-ray of the abdomen to see if a lump is visible.
- IVP (page 34): an X-ray to outline the kidneys. A Wilm's tumour usually distorts the structure of the kidney. Tomograms (page 44) may be done to get better views of the tumour.
- A chest X-ray is routinely done to make sure that there has been no spread to the lungs.

- If required, an arteriogram (page 41) may be done to outline the blood vessels in the kidney. This is a skilled procedure, especially in young babies, and should only be done by those experienced in doing the test in babies.
- An ultrasound (page 45) of the abdomen may be useful in showing up a lump.
- Abdominal CT scans (page 47) are being used more commonly.
- Liver ultrasound (page 45) or isotope scan (page 50).
- Lung tomograms (page 44) or CT scan (page 47) to look for small tumour nodules in the lungs.
- Bone scan (page 49) or bone X-ray.

This tumour may be confused with a neuroblastoma (page 229) of the adrenal gland, which lies just above the kidney, and a urine collection may be done to see if it contains catecholamines (page 230).

TREATMENT

The chances for cure of this common tumour are, fortunately, very good and because of this, and the complicated treatment necessary, children should be treated in a cancer centre.

The factors that affect the chance of cure are:

(1) Age. Children under 2 years of age do better.
(2) Stage. The less the tumour has spread the better.
(3) The appearance of the tumour under a microscope.

Surgery (Chapter 10)

The key to cure is complete removal of the tumour. This usually means taking out the affected kidney, an operation called a total nephrectomy. This operation should be done by an experienced paediatric surgeon as it needs careful planning and assessment of tumour spread. Many surgeons use metal clips to outline the site of the cancer in case radiotherapy is planned. Although in the past this operation was done as an emergency, it is much better to do it as a carefully planned procedure. If there are tumours affecting both kidneys it is often possible to remove the tumours and to leave enough unaffected kidney for the child to carry on a normal life. These children must be looked after by specialists, so that the very best operation can be planned.

Radiotherapy (Chapter 11)

Radiation is often used together with surgery and may be given before or after any operation. If radiotherapy is given before an operation it shrinks the cancer down and may makes its removal easier, but there are also advantages for doing the operation first. The radiotherapy must be carefully planned to avoid over-treating normal tissues, especially the bones of the spine. Treatment is given 4–5 days each week for about 3 weeks. The first visit to the radiotherapy department is spent in planning the treatment which is individualized for each child. Most children have the radiotherapy after an operation and this is started within 1 to 5 weeks. They tolerate the radiotherapy well as high doses are not used. If there are tumours of both kidneys then great care in planning radiation is needed.

Chemotherapy (Chapter 12)

On the whole these tumours respond well to drug treatment. Actinomycin D was the first drug to be used successfully and more recently cyclophosphamide, adriamycin and vincristine have been used. Chemotherapy is often started soon after an operation to remove the tumour and is then given intermittently for a period of up to 18 months. An idea of the side-effects of the drugs to be used can be seen from looking up the drugs in Appendix A. The drugs used and the frequency and length of time for which they are given may vary from hospital to hospital so discuss how this is to be done before treatment starts. Treatment is usually well tolerated apart from some sickness on the days when the drugs are given.

The total treatment plan must be designed for each individual case and it is not possible to give more than an outline of the typical methods of treatment. Although the treatment may seem complicated and to last for a long time most children are cured, so it is well worth it.

SUMMARY OF THE TREATMENT OF WILM'S TUMOUR

(1) The tumour is more common in some children with rare congenital abnormalities.

(2) Early symptoms are few and many children are only found to have a tumour when their parents notice a lump in their abdomen, often at bath-time.

(3) A carefully planned operation to remove all or as much of the tumour as possible is important.

(4) This may be followed by radiotherapy to the site of the cancer, though if it is a large tumour the radiotherapy may be used to shrink the cancer before an operation.

(5) Chemotherapy is used to treat any cancer cells that may have spread and is often started soon after the operation and is continued for up to 18 months.

(6) This is a tumour that can be cured and it should be treated in a special cancer centre. The cure rate is about 80 per cent and even children with very advanced Wilm's tumour or with tumour of both kidneys can be cured.

(7) The whole family needs the support of a specialist team.

CHAPTER 43

Soft tissue sarcomas

Soft tissue sarcomas are tumours of the soft parts of the body, and the commonest type (rhabdomyosarcoma) arises in muscles. The treatment of these uncommon tumours has improved markedly in the last two decades so that about half of the children with this tumour are cured. This improvement has come from the use of combinations of surgery, radiotherapy, and chemotherapy. No cause is known and it does not run in families except for rare inherited conditions that can become a sarcoma (for instance von Recklinghausen's disease, neurofibromatosis—page 6). Although most common in children these cancers can affect adults.

SYMPTOMS

This tumour can start in any part of the body but is most common in the head and neck, the arms or legs, and in the genito-urinary tract (page 000). Because of this the symptoms that it may cause vary according to the site of the tumour. The commonest symptom is swelling or a lump in a muscle. Though lumps and bruises are common and sarcomas are rare any child with a persistent lump in a muscle should be taken to a doctor. If a rhabdomyosarcoma or similar tumour is found the child should be treated in a specialist children's cancer centre.

DIAGNOSIS

A biopsy of the lump must be done to make sure of the diagnosis. Because these tumours tend to spread in lymphatics and the blood, a search must be made for metastases.

The following tests may be used:

- Bone scan (page 49) to check the bones.
- CT scan of the chest and abdomen (page 47).

- Liver scan (page 50) or ultrasound (page 45) to look for spread to the liver.
- Bone marrow biopsy (page 53). This is done under a general anaesthetic in children.

Other tests will depend on where the tumour has started. If this is in the genito-urinary tract then tests may include:

- An IVP (page 34) to outline the kidneys, ureters, and bladder.
- Barium enema (page 31) to see if anything is pressing on to the large bowel.

If the tumour involves the head and neck, extra information can be gained from the following tests.

- X-ray of the skull to see if the bones of the skull are involved.
- Brain scan (page 52), CT scan (page 47) to check whether there is any spread inside the skull.
- Lumbar puncture (page 252) to check that there is no involvement of the fluid around the brain (CSF).

TREATMENT

Frequently surgery, radiotherapy, and chemotherapy are all used together to try to cure the child. Though the treatment is complex and difficult to tolerate, children are more resilient than adults and the 50 per cent chance of cure makes the side-effects worthwhile. Because these tumours can grow in so many different parts of the body it is not possible to give a definite pattern of treatment and the next sections only outline the general type of therapy that is used.

Surgery (Chapter 10)

The initial treatment consists of surgical removal of as much of the tumour as possible. The chances of doing this will depend on where the tumour is, but every attempt is made to leave normal tissue and to get as good a cosmetic result as possible. Detailed discussion of the type of operation is beyond the scope of this book as it must be individualized for each child; parents must talk to the surgeon prior to any operation, as extensive surgery including amputation may be necessary.

Radiotherapy (Chapter 11)

Radiotherapy is often given to the tumour bed after as much as possible has been removed by an operation. High doses of radiotherapy may be required and treatment is divided into fractions given 4–5 days a week for 4 to 8 weeks. The side-effects of this treatment will, of course, depend on several factors and before treatment starts parents should discuss the proposed programme and its side-effects. An idea of these may be gained from Chapter 11. In some cases radiotherapy may be given before surgery in an attempt to make it possible to remove a tumour.

Chemotherapy (Chapter 12)

Chemotherapy is often combined with local treatment either to deal with cancer that is known to have spread, or to treat suspected metastases even when none can be found (adjuvant treatment).

The drugs most commonly used are a combination of the following:

(1) Actinomycin D.
(2) Vinctristine.
(3) Cyclophosphamide.
(4) Adriamycin.

A combination of these drugs is usually given at 3-weekly intervals. The duration of treatment depends on whether the drugs are being given for metastatic disease or as an adjuvant for suspected disease. Parents will need to discuss the possible side-effects of treatment though most children are able to tolerate treatment better than adults. An idea of the toxicity of each of the drugs in a combination can be gained from looking up the individual drugs in Appendix A.

OUTLOOK

This depends on several factors.

• Site. Tumours developing in some parts of the body do

comparatively better; these include tumours of the bladder, female genital tract, and around the eye.

- Stage. The chance of cure is clearly best in those with a small tumour that has not spread.
- Appearance under a microscope. The pattern the tumour forms varies and some (embryonal and botryoid) tumours do better than others.
- Age. Some studies have suggested that younger children have the best chance of cure.

SUMMARY OF THE TREATMENT OF SOFT TISSUE SARCOMAS

(1) These tumours can affect may different parts of the body.
(2) Treatment and its side-effects vary according to where the tumour is.
(3) At operation an attempt is made to remove all or as much as possible of the tumour and extensive surgery may be needed in some cases. Parents need to discuss the type of surgery and its consequences in detail.
(4) Radiotherapy must be used with surgery to treat the site of the tumour. High doses are often needed and these may cause side-effects and parents should discuss these. Radiotherapy may be given before or after an operation.
(5) Drug therapy (chemotherapy) is often given after local treatment. This may be given even if there is no evidence of disease spread, as there is often a high risk of microscopic deposits of tumour that cannot be seen. Chemotherapy causes side-effects which need to be discussed before treatment.
(6) Despite the intensive type of treatments used for these tumours most children will tolerate the treatment reasonably well.
(7) The whole family will need the support of their own doctor and of a team of specialists during and after the treatment.
(8) This is a tumour that should be treated in a specialist cancer centre.

CHAPTER 44

Chondrosarcoma

Unlike many of the bone tumours, chondrosarcomas often occur in middle life as well as in children. They tend to be slow-growing and spread late in their course so that surgical removal is often curative. Some develop from pre-existing benign bone tumours called osteochondromas, enchondromas, or chondromas.

They can grow anywhere and staging is mainly concerned with the extent of the primary tumour. The tests used include, plain X-rays, CT scans (page 47), and sometimes arteriograms (page 41).

TREATMENT

This is almost exclusively surgical. Most often the tumour and some surrounding bone are removed and this is all that is necessary. Occasionally if the tumour is large an amputation may be necessary. Surgery for this tumour should be done by someone experienced in the field as a common error is inadequate removal of the cancer.

CHAPTER 45

Ewing's sarcoma

Ewing's sarcoma is a malignant tumour of bones that is most common between the ages of 5 and 16 years. Almost any bone can be involved and the tumour is more common in boys. It can rarely occur in adults and outside bones.

SYMPTOMS

As with other bone cancers the common symptoms are:

- Increasing and persistent pain over a bone.
- Swelling over bone.
- Decrease in movement if a limb bone is involved.

DIAGNOSIS

An X-ray will often show a swollen bone with an area of destruction. It is not always possible to be sure if this is a tumour, infection or another disease. Because of this a biopsy (sample of a small piece of tissue) is always necessary.

If a cancer is suspected other investigations will include:

- A chest X-ray to make sure there has been no spread to the lungs. Lung tomograms (page 44) or a CT scan (page 47) may be done.
- A bone scan (page 49) or X-rays of other bones to see if the cancer has spread.
- A liver ultrasound (page 45) or isotope scan (page 50) may be used to examine the liver.
- A bone marrow biopsy (page 53) may be performed (under anaesthetic) to check for spread.

TREATMENT

As with most cancers in children a team of doctors is involved and children should be treated at a special cancer centre.

Surgery (Chapter 10)

The most important role of surgery in this tumour is to obtain a small piece (a biopsy) for microscopic examination. This is crucial to make the diagnosis and so that further treatment can be planned. The biopsy is usually taken from tumour in the soft tissue around the bone and is very rarely disfiguring. In most cases no further operation is needed though in certain parts of the body where it is difficult to cure the tumour with radiotherapy and drugs the place of an operation is being tested.

It is sometimes difficult to tell a Ewing's sarcoma from other tumours and pathologists may need to do special tests or to send the tissue biopsied to other pathologists. Because of this it may take some days to get an answer from the biopsy.

Radiotherapy (Chapter 11)

This is usually the most important treatment. However, very high doses of radiation are needed and this treatment should only be given by experienced radiotherapists. Because of the high doses of radiotherapy it is important that a programme of active exercises is used during and after treatment to make sure that the function of the area treated is as good as possible. The first visit to the radiotherapy department is spent planning the individual treatment. The radiotherapy is then given for 4–5 days per week for 6–8 weeks. The immediate side-effects of treatment include soreness and reddening of the irradiated skin; this cannot be avoided because of the high dose being used and loose fitting clothes should be worn to avoid rubbing the skin. After radiotherapy, gradual thickening or scarring (fibrosis) of the skin occurs and unless physiotherapy exercises are conscientiously used poor movement of joints can result.

Chemotherapy (Chapter 12)

Radiotherapy is used to eradicate the local tumour, whereas drugs are used to treat cancer cells that have spread to other parts of the body. This is a very malignant tumour that frequently spreads and even if all tests are normal, treatment is given for hidden disease (microscopic or micro-metastases). The drugs that are most often used are vincristine, cyclo-phosphamide, adriamycin, and actinomycin D. Treatment is given intermittently for some months and parents will need to discuss the type and duration of treatment before it starts.

The nature of combined radiotherapy–chemotherapy treatment will depend on several factors and treatment will have to be planned for each child. Radiotherapy may also be used locally to treat a tumour that has already spread to other parts of the body. The chances of cure have increased with modern management but, unfortunately, less than half the children treated will survive this tumour.

SUMMARY OF THE TREATMENT OF EWING'S SARCOMA

(1) This tumour of bones can arise anywhere.
(2) Surgery is usually only done to make the diagnosis.
(3) High doses of radiotherapy are used together with chemotherapy.
(4) The cure rate has risen from 10 per cent to 40–50 per cent.
(5) Treatment should be given in a specialist centre.
(6) The whole family need the help and support of an experienced team.

CHAPTER 46

Osteogenic sarcoma

This tumour of bone is most common between the ages of 10 and 25 years and is more prevalent in boys. Any bones in the body can be involved but the limb bones are most frequently affected.

SYMPTOMS

Pain and swelling of the involved part together with reduction in the use of the limb are the usual symptoms. There is often a tender lump and occasionally weight loss and malaise occur. Sometimes a weakened bone may break—a pathological fracture. Spread of the tumour is common and the lungs and other bones are most often involved.

DIAGNOSIS

An X-ray of the bone will usually show an area of destruction and thickening which may be typical for this tumour. If an X-ray shows this type of abnormality the child should be referred to a specialist cancer centre.

A sample of bone (biopsy) must be taken to make the diagnosis and before this is done more X-rays may be necessary. If the biopsy does show an oesteogenic sarcoma, then further tests are used to see if the tumour has spread. The tests include:

- Chest X-ray.
- Lung tomograms (page 44) or CT scan (page 47) to examine the lungs in greater detail.
- Bone scan (page 49).
- Liver scan (page 50) or ultrasound (page 45).

TREATMENT

The treatment of this tumour has changed markedly in the past ten years. Before the 1970s surgery was the main treatment, but despite amputations tumour developed in the lungs within a few months and the child died. This was due to hidden cancer cells (micro- and microscopic metastases) in other parts of the body. Because of this, treatment now includes chemotherapy and/or radiotherapy.

Surgery (Chapter 10)

Because most tumours start in a limb, bone operations in the past usually meant removal of the affected part of the limb (an amputation). Though this sounds rather drastic it may be the only way of being sure of getting rid of the cancer and often gives the best chance of survival. Recently, in certain cases, cancer centres have been testing whether extensive surgery (but not amputation) together with radiotherapy is as good as amputation. This is an experimental approach only available in special centres, and although it usually means that the limb is saved a series of operations may be necessary and the limb is unlikely to function entirely normally. Parents must discuss the type of surgery recommended and its consequences in great detail. If an amputation is necessary it must be remembered that all these children will adapt well to an artificial limb and will, in most respects, be able to live a normal life. A programme of intensive rehabilitation should always be planned from the outset and can only be done by those experienced in this area of medicine. Some studies comparing amputation with extensive limb-sparing surgery have shown that children undergoing amputation adjusted better to the disability caused by surgery.

Radiotherapy (Chapter 11)

Some centres use high doses of radiotherapy to shrink a tumour before an operation designed to preserve the limb. This type of treatment remains experimental and the effects of extensive surgery and radiation may mean that the limb does not work well.

Chemotherapy (Chapter 12)

Most centres use combinations of chemotherapy drugs before or after surgery and/or radiotherapy. This is because of the very high risk of tumour spread (even if the usual tests are normal). The drugs most frequently used are methotrexate, adriamycin, vincristine, and cyclophosphamide and an idea of the side-effects of a regime can be gained from looking up the individual drugs in Appendix A. Treatment is usually given intermittently for 1 to 2 years and children usually feel sick and unwell for a few days with each treatment. Young children tolerate this well but teenagers find it is more difficult. Recent clinical trials show that such 'adjuvant' therapy does increase the chances of cure.

If there is metastatic spread of the cancer, chemotherapy is used; but surgical removal of tumour lumps (often from the lungs) is becoming more common and is curative in some cases.

OUTLOOK

The chances for cure have improved in the past 10 years from about 15 per cent to 40–50 per cent.

The factors affecting the prognosis are:

- Stage when diagnosed—the outlook is poor if there are already metastases.
- The microscopic appearance—a particular type of osteogenic sarcoma (paraosteal) is slower-growing and 70–80 per cent of these patients are cured by an amputation alone.

SUMMARY OF THE TREATMENT OF OSTEOGENIC SARCOMA

(1) This is the commonest type of bone cancer and is most often seen between the ages of 10 and 25 years.
(2) Pain, swelling, and reduced movement of a limb are the most common symptoms.
(3) Investigations are done to see if the tumour has spread and a biopsy of the tumour must be done to confirm the diagnosis.
(4) Treatment should be in a special children's cancer centre.
(5) Amputation is the standard treatment but radiotherapy

and/or chemotherapy may be used before an operation to preserve the limb; such an approach remains experimental.

(6) Intensive rehabilitation must be planned from the outset.

(7) Most centres use chemotherapy before or after surgery.

(8) Paraosteal sarcomas are slow-growing and are usually curable with an amputation.

(9) Metastases are sometimes removed surgically (usually from the lungs) and such operations together with chemotherapy can be curative.

(10) The chances of cure have risen from 15 per cent to 40–50 per cent.

(11) The whole family need the help and support of a full team of specialists.

CHAPTER 47

Leukaemia

Leukaemia is cancer of the bone marrow cells, and in the past decade there have been great improvements in its treatment. There are several different types of leukaemia but only one of these, acute lymphocytic leukaemia (ALL), is common in children.

Acute lymphocytic leukaemia is, in fact, the commonest type of cancer in children, accounting for about one-third of all childhood cancers. It is usually seen between the ages of 2 and 7 years and is uncommon after the age of 15.

As leukaemia is a cancer that grows in the bone marrow, where blood is made, the leukaemic cells make it difficult for the body to form new blood. Because of this children become short of red cells (anaemic), white cells (becoming susceptible to infections), and the clotting cells called platelets (making them prone to bleeding).

SYMPTOMS

To begin with these are non-specific and include:

- Tiredness.
- Frequent infections that do not respond normally to antibiotics.
- Occasionally pain over the spleen (left side of abdomen).

Further symptoms that often develop are:

- Bruising, bleeding (particularly from the gums and nose), a rash consisting of tiny bleeding spots in the skin (petechiae or purpura).
- Enlargement of lymph glands (page 23).
- Discovery of a lump in the abdomen (an enlarged spleen).
- Pain or discomfort over bones.

DIAGNOSIS

If leukaemia is suspected a routine blood count should be taken. When leukaemia is found the count is usually abnormal. The changes in the count include:

- Anaemia (lack of red cells).
- A low white count due to a loss of normal cells, or a high white count because of leukaemic cells present in the blood.
- Lack of platelets (thrombocytopenia).

Although these abnormalities may strongly suggest leukaemia a bone marrow test (page 53) should always be done. In young children this is often done under a general anaesthetic and is best performed by those experienced in the treatment of leukaemia in children.

TREATMENT

Ideally all children with leukaemia (ALL) should be treated in a special children's cancer centre. This is a curable disease and every effort should be made to cure the child. The first stage of treatment is called 'remission induction'.

Remission induction

The first object of treatment is to get rid of all the leukaemic cells in the body. Drug treatment (chemotherapy) is used and two drugs, vincristine and prednisone, are the mainstay of treatment. They have far fewer side-effects than the types of treatment used for adult leukaemia. The major problem that children may notice is some 'pins and needles' in the fingers or feet; this is caused by vincristine and goes away after the treatment is stopped. During this early period of treatment children are at risk from infection or bleeding and must be watched closely. They may need to be in hospital during induction though most hospitals make every effort to get children home as soon as possible. Support with blood transfusions, antibiotics, and platelets transfusions may be needed to treat anaemia, infections, and bleeding respectively.

Over 90 per cent of children will be in complete remission (page 259) within one month. This does not mean they are cured, only that the leukaemia has been reduced to such an extent that it cannot be detected. All tests during a complete remission are normal and the child will feel much better. For the small proportion of children not in complete remission further treatment with other drugs is given.

Induction treatment for this type of leukaemia is, therefore, very successful and well tolerated though the child must be watched carefully for infection or bleeding. As soon as the child is in complete remission (CR) more treatment must be given to the brain and spinal cord.

Central nervous system prophylaxis

In the past, up to half of children in complete remission developed leukaemia of the lining (meninges) of the brain and spinal cord. Because of this, treatment is given to prevent its occurrence (central nervous system prophylaxis) and is now an essential part of the treatment of childhood leukaemia. The treatment consists of radiotherapy to the head and a course of about five injections into the fluid in the spine (an intrathecal injection). Radiotherapy (Chapter 11) is given about 4–5 times a week for about two weeks and causes *temporary* hair loss but is well tolerated. The intrathecal injections of a drug called methotrexate may be given under a general anaesthetic in young children, but should not be painful if performed skilfully. The combination of brain radiotherapy and intrathecal injections may cause temporary sleepiness but there are usually no obvious long-term effects. Because there is a risk of leukaemia in the testis, some hospitals give radiotherapy to the testicles to try to prevent this. This remains experimental but will always cause sterility. After the child has achieved a complete remission and has had CNS prophylactic treatment, further chemotherapy, called maintenance therapy, is given.

Maintenance therapy

This usually consists of two or more drugs given by mouth in moderate doses. This is to remove any remaining microscopic collections of leukaemic cells. The doses are chosen so that they are well tolerated and the child is able to return to a normal life style.

However, regular blood counts are required to monitor the treatment and adjustments of the drug doses may be needed. Bone marrow examinations may be done every so often to check that all remains normal. The period of maintenance is usually at least 2 years and if the child has remained in complete remission all of this time the treatment is stopped altogether.

Viewed all at once the remission induction, CNS prophylaxis, and maintenance therapy seems a heavy programme for a child to cope with, but if the treatment is completed the chance of cure is good.

Infection remains one of the problems throughout the treatment period. Any child undergoing treatment for leukaemia who develops signs of an infection should be seen by a doctor. These children do not have normal defence mechanisms and they respond badly to common infections, such as measles, and are more prone to unusual infections.

It is very important to try to protect these children from the common viral illnesses of childhood, such as chickenpox, which may cause a fatal pneumonia in children being treated for leukaemia. Leukaemic children should live a normal life but must be isolated from friends and family who have an infection. Injections of immune serum can be given to children exposed to chickenpox infection but it is better to avoid contact with the infection. Prompt and expert treatment of any infection that does occur is important and most children will, with appropriate treatment, recover.

RELAPSE

If the leukaemia returns it is said to have relapsed. It is usually possible to give further remission induction therapy and obtain a complete remission for a second, third, or even fourth time. However, the length of the remission gradually becomes shorter and few children with recurrent leukaemia live more than a few years. Recently, children relapsing with ALL are being considered for a bone marrow transplantation and this may offer a small chance of cure.

SUPPORT

In addition to expertise in treating leukaemia a children's cancer centre can provide the emotional and practical support that is most important for the family of the child with leukaemia. The period of treatment is long and fraught with difficulty and even with complete remission the future is uncertain. This is difficult for parents and hard to come to terms with, but with experienced medical staff problems can be recognized and discussed and appropriate support given.

THE CHANCES OF CURE

About half of all patients with childhood acute lymphocytic leukaemia can be cured with current treatment. The risk of relapse is highest in the two years after stopping treatment and the risk then gets progressively less. This greatly improved chance of cure has only come from the careful use of all the treatments described.

SUMMARY OF THE TREATMENT OF CHILDHOOD ACUTE LYMPHOCYTIC LEUKAEMIA

(1) The commonest symptoms are of tiredness, infections, bleeding, and enlarged lymph nodes.
(2) The first stage of treatment is remission induction. Vincristine and prednisone are usually used and the treatment is well tolerated.
(3) The child may need hospitalization for part of this period.
(4) Over 90 per cent of children have a complete remission.
(5) The next step is CNS prophylaxis. Radiotherapy is given to the brain together with a course of intrathecal injections.
(6) Following this, two or more years maintenance drug therapy is given. Infections are a risk during maintenance.
(7) If there has been no relapse, treatment is then stopped. The subsequent risk of relapse is highest in the first two years after treatment.
(8) The chance of cure is about 50 per cent.

CHAPTER 48

Lymphomas

The treatment and outlook for children with lymphoma is different from that of adults.

HODGKIN'S DISEASE

The risk of Hodgkin's disease is very low in babies but gradually rises in childhood to reach a peak in the twenties. The spread of this disease and its staging is the same as in adults (page 179). The investigations used to find out the extent of the disease include:

- Chest X-ray and possibly lung tomograms (page 44).
- Lymphangiogram (page 38).
- Full blood count and biochemical tests on the blood.
- Bone marrow examination (page 53).
- Liver and bone scans (pages 50 and 49).

In adults an exploratory operation including removal of the spleen (staging laparotomy—page 181) is usually carried out in patients being considered for radiotherapy rather than chemotherapy. However, children are usually treated with a combination of radiotherapy and chemotherapy and the operation is less important. Many hospitals do not, therefore, use a staging laparotomy and will go straight ahead with combined therapy. The chances of cure are good with this cancer but are affected by the stage, as in adults.

TREATMENT

It is important to avoid giving a large dose of radiotherapy to growing bones and for this reason low doses are used together with chemotherapy even in patients with apparently localized disease. This has the added advantage that a staging laparotomy is not needed. This is useful because there is a risk of infection after removal of the spleen. A treatment plan will be designed for each child and parents will need to discuss the details of the treatment before it starts. The chapters on radiotherapy, chemotherapy, and adult Hodgkin's disease will suggest some questions and the following list may be helpful.

(1) Is a staging laparotomy being considered?
(2) Is radiotherapy or chemotherapy or a combination of both to be used.
(3) What are the immediate side-effects of treatment?
(4) How long will the treatment take?
(5) Are there any long-term effects of treatment?
(6) Does the treatment affect fertility?
(7) What are the chances of cure?

As with all childhood cancers it is desirable that the child should be treated in a special centre.

NON-HODGKIN'S LYMPHOMA

As in adults there are numerous different types of non-Hodgkin's lymphoma. However, most fall into the group of more rapidly growing and potentially curable lymphomas.

Symptoms

Children can develop many different symptoms but several groups of symptoms are typical.

- Tumour in the chest, around the heart may cause shortness of breath, swollen glands in the neck, and fluid in the chest (a pleural effusion—page 275). There may be involvement of the bone marrow.
- Disease in the digestive tract. The small bowel and stomach are most frequently involved. Children may develop stoppages of the bowel (bowel obstruction) and the diagnosis of lymphoma is often only made at an operation to find the cause of obstruction.
- Disease of lymph nodes in the abdomen. Children may develop greatly enlarged abdominal lymph nodes which can be felt as lumps. There may be no obvious disease outside

the abdomen and an exploratory operation (a laparotomy) may be needed to make the diagnosis.

- Enlarged lymph nodes. Other children may develop enlarged nodes in the neck, groin, or under the arms. Often the nodes are confined to one of these areas.

- Tonsil or adenoid involvement. Lymphoma of these glands is often associated with enlarged lymph nodes in the neck. Occasionally it is associated with involvement of the stomach or bowel.

Investigation and treatment

Because of the differing patterns of spread and of types of lymphoma it is too complicated to give more than an outline of treatment.

Investigations will vary from child to child but may include:

- Chest X-ray.
- Lymphangiogram (page 38).
- Full blood count and biochemical tests on the blood.
- Bone marrow examination (page 53).
- Liver and bone scans (pages 50 and 49).
- An explanatory operation may be needed to make the diagnosis in cases of bowel obstruction or in disease confined to the abdomen.

Treatment varies from hospital to hospital but will be based on common principles. Because most of these lymphomas are of a fast-growing type, the treatment is intensive with several drugs (combination chemotherapy) to eradicate all traces of the cancer. This may be combined with radiation therapy and is often followed by a period of less intensive maintenance chemotherapy (see Chapter 47 page 250) for up to two years. There is also an increased risk of lymphoma of the lining of the brain with certain types of childhood lymphoma and prophylactic X-ray therapy and drugs (page 252) may be needed, as in leukaemic children. The treatment is often complicated and the side-effects and duration of treatment may seem formidable, but the good chance of cure makes it worthwhile. As in leukaemia, families need total support during treatment and care in a special children's cancer centre is preferable.

SUMMARY OF THE TREATMENT OF CHILDHOOD LYMPHOMA

(1) There are several types of lymphoma in children. Most are fast-growing.

(2) There are several patterns of lymphoma, including spread in the chest, stomach or bowel, lymph nodes in the abdomen, lymph nodes in the rest of the body, and lymphoma of the tonsils.

(3) Investigations are done to 'stage' the disease. An exploratory abdominal operation may be needed to make the diagnosis in some children.

(4) Treatment mainly uses chemotherapy though radiotherapy may also be used in certain children.

(5) In some lymphomas, treatment may be given to prevent spread to the brain.

(6) If a complete remission is achieved, maintenance treatment is often given for about two years.

(7) For some children the chance of cure is good.

CHAPTER 49

What are response, relapse and remission?

Medical language is hard to follow; this chapter aims to explain some of the terms used when talking about the way a cancer responds to treatment and how well patients do.

RESPONSE OR REMISSION

These words are used to describe a reduction in the size of tumour. The proportion (per cent) of patients who achieve a response is called the response rate. Responses may be of two main types.

- Partial response or remission (PR) is defined as a reduction in the size of a 'measurable' tumour that is greater than half (50 per cent) and lasts for at least one month. There is, however, still detectable tumour. Shrinkage of tumour that is less than half is usually disregarded by doctors as not being useful. The partial response rate is the proportion of patients whose tumour shrinks to less than half of its previous size.
- Complete response or remission (CR). This is complete disappearance of a tumour so that it is not detectable on examination or after repeating all tests that were previously abnormal. Occasionally, as in ovarian cancer (page 135), there may be a second operation to ensure that there is no remaining tumour. A complete remission does **not** mean cure. It only indicates that there is no tumour that can be seen using our present-day tests. If there are even a few surviving cancer cells then they may grow back so that the tumour eventually reappears. The complete response rate is the proportion of patients achieving a complete remission.
- Overall response rate is a term used to combine the partial and complete responders. It is the proportion of patients who

have a complete response or shrinkage of their tumour by at least a half.

RELAPSE

A patient who has gained a complete remission then has the tumour grow back is said to have relapsed. Relapse does not imply that further treatment is not helpful and in some cancers a second complete remission and cure is still possible.

PROGRESSION

Progression is a term implying that a tumour has continued to grow despite treatment. It may also be used to describe a tumour which starts to grow again after a partial response.

SURVIVAL

When treatments are being tested in trials, the length of time that patients survive is often quoted. The figure that is usually given is the length of time that has elapsed when half the patients have died. This is called the *median survival* time.

Information on survival should be related to the important factors that are known to influence the patient's outlook. However, doctors can never give an accurate estimate of how long a patient will live as everybody is different. Most doctors will be reluctant to say how a patient will do, and any figure given must only be taken as approximate.

RELAPSE-FREE SURVIVAL (PROGRESSION FREE INTERVAL)

This is a term that only applies to patients who achieve a complete remission. It is the time from the start of treatment till the disease relapses.

CURE

It may seem odd that it is difficult to define cure. The proper definition is that the survival of a group of patients is the same as a similar group of people who do not have the cancer that is being studied. In other words, the patients with cancer die of other diseases at the same rate as a normal population. This definition can never be usefully applied as it takes very many years to gather such information.

Instead, cure is usually talked about in terms of lack of tumour *relapse* over a defined period of time. Although there are often no clear guidelines, this period of time varies from tumour to tumour. Thus, in the case of testicular teratomas a two-year period without relapse is regarded by many cancer specialists as tantamount to cure. For Hodgkin's disease a five-year period is required, whilst in breast cancer relapses can occur after ten years and a fifteen- or twenty-year period may be necessary before cure can be talked about. Despite this, it is true of all cancers that the risk of relapse is greatest in the first year after stopping treatment and with each succeeding year the risk diminishes.

CHAPTER 50

Treatment for the symptoms of cancer

Cancer may cause all sorts of different symptoms depending on which part of the body it affects. As well as specific treatment to reduce or get rid of the tumour other treatments can be used to reduce the symptoms. Both approaches should be used together, though in very advanced cases it may be best to rely on treatment of the symptoms only.

Because anticancer treatment often causes side-effects (Chapters 10 to 12) it is sometimes necessary to use other drugs to try to reduce these effects. Treatment of symptoms is, therefore, very important.

PAIN CONTROL

Most people associate cancer with a painful progressive illness that ends in death. In fact about one-half of patients with *advanced* cancers have no significant pain. For those patients who do have pain, expert care is important.

One of the most important reasons for failure to control pain is a lack of appreciation by doctors that it is not a simple physical sensation. As well as the physical perception of pain there is an emotional reaction to it. Perception of pain and pain thresholds are, therefore, closely linked to mood and morale and a good relationship between patient and doctor is very helpful.

Pain is extremely difficult to evaluate. It varies from person to person; some can tolerate a lot more than others without requesting relief. It is hard to describe: 'like toothache', a 'stab-bing feeling', a 'sharp pain', a 'dull ache'. It is even difficult to sometimes point to exactly where the pain is: a good guide for doctors evaluating cancer pain is that 'the pain is what the patient says it is'. Pain-killers are especially helpful and the right dose, to ensure complete relief without causing drowsiness, needs expert care. Patients should work together with their doctor to achieve the best control.

Description of pain

It is very difficult to describe the quality of a pain, though descriptions like 'a gnawing toothache' or 'a stabbing pain' can be helpful. Because it may be difficult for a patient to say exactly where a pain is, it may be useful to draw in the area of pain on a picture of the body.

Pain often varies in intensity during the day, though this may be due to the use of inadequate drugs which only ease pain for an hour or so, allowing pain to return before the next dose. Pain at night may be worse than during the day as people are more likely to feel alone at this time and may not take pain-killers at night. If a pain is worse on movement or weight-bearing tell your doctor.

A pain may be chronic or acute. Chronic pain can become all-consuming and it:

- Has no foreseeable end.
- Tends to get worse not better.
- Serves no purpose.
- Takes up all of one's attention and makes life not worth living.

Such pain requires expert treatment and in most cases it is possible to control it and make life worthwhile again.

Use of pain-killing drugs (analgesics)

The key to successfully controlling pain is to make sure that it is kept at bay *all* the time. For this reason it is wrong to delay taking a pain medicine until the pain has come back and is bad again. Continuous pain logically requires continuous treatment, so regular doses of drugs which prevent the pain returning should be used. Some doctors still prescribe pain-killers 'to be taken as required'—this is not helpful, except in intermittent pain, as the drug *must* be taken before the pain returns. If after taking a pain-killer you are pain-free for 4 to 5 hours then you will need your next tablet after about 3½ hours. Most pain-killers work for approximately 4 hours if given in the correct dose.

Pain at night can be a problem and sometimes it is better to set an alarm clock to wake you in the middle of the night for the next dose rather than be woken by pain a little later and not get back to sleep. Once pain has returned it takes longer to get under control and often increasing doses of pain-killers are needed. Although many people and even doctors worry about taking medicines, regular and adequate doses of pain-killers are essential and safe if used correctly. Doctors are more and more aware of this and so the standard of pain control has improved in the past ten years.

Choice of pain-killer

This depends on the severity of the pain and treatment starts with the simplest drug likely to be useful.

(1) Mild pain

This can be controlled by aspirin or paracetamol (Panadol). Regular use of 1 or 2 tablets every 4–6 hours is recommended and many patients can tolerate up to 4 tablets of aspirin every 4 hours. However, patients receiving chemotherapy or those with a low blood count should try to avoid aspirin as it damages the platelets (page 80).

(2) Moderate pain

When aspirin and paracetamol fail, then weak narcotic drugs are used. A combination of drugs including a codeine derivative is often used. The commonly used drugs (brand names) include:

(1) Distalgesic (containing paracetamol and dextro-propoxyphene).
(2) Napsalgesic (containing aspirin and dextropropoxyphene).
(3) Codis (containing aspirin and codeine phosphate).
(4) Paracodal (containing paracetamol and codeine).
(5) DF118 (containing dihydrocodeine tartrate).

(6) Paramol–118 (containing paracetamol and dihydrocodeine tartrate).

The usual dose is 1 or 2 tablets taken regularly every 4–6 hours.

(3) Severe pain

This requires much stronger drugs and narcotics are usually given. These are a group of opium-like substances that are powerful pain-killers. When used for severe pain, they do not result in drug addiction or dependence. Unfortunately, many patients, nurses, and doctors do not realize this. It is always worth using these drugs when pain is severe and often the dose can be reduced once the pain is controlled. There are various ways of giving narcotic drugs and several preparations. It is nearly always best to give the drug by mouth though injections may be better for a few patients. The preparations that are available include:

(1) Nepenthe (with or without aspirin): a mixture of opium alkaloids with a measured amount of morphine.

(2) Morphine syrup ⎫ these may be mixed with
(3) Diamorphine syrup ⎬ alcohol or a fruit drink and
　　　　　　　　　　⎭ only differ in potency.

(4) MST: a slow-release morphine in a special tablet.
(5) Buprenorphine: a new pain-killer for moderate pain.

Other drugs (brand names) similar in strength can be used.

(6) Palfium: potent but short-acting.
(7) Narphen: a potent alternative to diamorphine less likely to cause nausea—not available as a liquid.
(8) Dromoran: a potent short-acting alternative.

These strong drugs cannot be bought at a chemist's shop and can only be prescribed by a doctor.

Overwhelming pain is rare, but requires urgent medical treatment and the most effective way of dealing with such pain is to give injections of a narcotic pain-killer (usually diamorphine) together with a sedative such as valium. This can be repeated, with increasing doses, every 1 to 2 hours until the pain is controlled. The patient, who will be exhaused anyway, may then sleep for long periods and when the pain has been controlled for several days the doses may be reduced and the drugs given less frequently by mouth.

This is not an exhaustive list of pain drugs and many patients may be given different drugs and it should be remembered that the drug names may vary by country. It is also worth knowing that most drugs have a proper name and a drug company (proprietary) name.

Whichever drugs are used it is the regular use of the pain-killer *before* pain returns that is paramount.

Other drugs that may be used together with pain-killers

Various drugs useful for anxiety or depression may be added to pain-killers. This helps by reducing the psychological part of the pain as well as by increasing the power of the pain-killer. The drugs (proprietary names) that may be used include:

(1) Largactil (chlorpromazine)
(2) Valium and other anti-anxiety drugs.
(3) Many different antidepressants.
(4) Sleeping tablets at night.

Steroids can also be beneficial and prednisolone or dexamethasone tablets may be given with pain-killers for certain specific pains. In addition they often have a non-specific effect of making patients feel better, increase appetite, and lift mood. Drugs usually used for rheumatic conditions (anti-inflammatory drugs) may also be given with pain-killers, especially if the pain is in a bone or caused by pressure on a nerve.

Other ways of controlling pain

(1) Pain sensations are carried by nerves and it is often possible to stop (block) the nerve from carrying the pain impulses to the brain. This can be done by injecting a long-acting local anaesthetic near to the nerve (as a dentist does) or by using an injection which damages the nerve permanently. These techniques are specialized and patients need to discuss their use, but they should be available in most general

hospitals. They are often less useful for cancer pain than for chronic pain of other causes.

(2) Hypnosis is only an adjunct to other methods of treating pain. It produces an altered state of consciousness, even in difficult subjects, and helps them to control their own pain. Whilst this may be successful in some patients it is not commonly used; often its great value is that a doctor will spend half an hour with you.

(3) Acupuncture. Though this would seem, by anecdote, to be a useful treatment, it remains to be tested in cancer patients. Its disadvantage is that the effect does not last long.

(4) Peripheral nerve stimulation. Electrical stimulation of the skin near painful areas may reduce pain. This is most effective if the result lasts after the stimulation has stopped.

(5) Nitrous oxide gas mixtures. Very severe short-lasting pains are difficult to deal with and some hospitals get patients to breathe an anaesthetic gas mixture, nitrous oxide, when they get a spasm of pain. The effect comes on quickly and passes off quickly and it may occasionally be useful for short but severe pains, e.g. if turning in bed hurts or changing a dressing causes discomfort.

The control of pain is complex and severe pain often needs the help of a doctor skilled in this field. Important points to remember are:

- Pain is not only physical—every effort should be made to deal with anxiety and depression. Tell people how you feel if you want to.
- If drugs are used, take them regularly so that the pain does not return between doses.
- If pain is severe, narcotic drugs are needed; these will not cause addiction.
- Other methods of pain control are available.
- Substantial pain control can almost always be achieved.

CONSTIPATION

Constipation can be more troublesome than pain for patients with cancer. It is probably due to change in diet, loss of appetite, chemotherapy, depression, unaccustomed inactivity perhaps,

and most importantly, the use of pain-killing drugs. It is important to consider ways of dealing with this and doctors will
probably recommend a laxative, which with sensible use will
help.

Laxatives may be of several types:

(1) Purgatives, such as senna, that work by stimulating the
    bowel.
(2) Stool softeners, such as liquid paraffin and drugs that
    increase the bulk.
(3) Other drugs, such as Dorbanex Medro, are a combination
    of these drugs and work both ways. If purgatives are given
    alone they may cause colicky pain and it is usually best to
    give a stool softener as well. If, after 3 days, laxatives
    have failed to work, then further treatment is required and
    suppositories are commonly used, though it may become
    necessary to give an enema.

When narcotic pain-killers are used laxatives should always
be used to prevent constipation.

DIARRHOEA

This may be a symptom of the cancer or a side-effect of its
treatment. The best antidiarrhoeal drug is codeine phosphate (1
or 2 tablets, three times a day). Other drugs are also effective
and they can be used together in severe cases and act by prolonging bowel transit and increasing fluid absorption.

NAUSEA AND VOMITING

This may be caused by the cancer but is also very common
after chemotherapy (Chapter 12) and radiotherapy (Chapter 11).
If nausea and vomiting is severe it may be necessary to start
treatment with injections of antisickness drugs (antiemetics) as
any pills will be vomited back. Alternatively, suppositories may
be used.

Drugs used include the following (trade name in brackets):

Chlorpramazine (Largactil)
Prochlorperazine (Stemetil)
Promazine (Sparine) } acting mainly on the brain
Cyclizine (Marzine)
Dexamethasone (Decadrone)
Metoclopramide (Maxolon)—acting mainly on the bowel.

They may be used alone or in combination since they act in different parts of the body or brain. It is most difficult to prevent the vomiting caused by anticancer chemotherapy and new antisickness drugs are being tested. Most antisickness drugs can be used every 4–6 hours and the next tablet should be taken before the sickness returns. Because they may cause drowsiness, avoid driving whilst on these drugs.

LOSS OF APPETITE

Loss of appetite and weight is very common with all sorts of cancer and may be due to several factors:

(1) Poor appetite causing a reduction in intake of calories and protein.
(2) The tumour altering the body's metabolism and 'burning' up excessive amounts of energy.
(3) Symptoms of the cancer (or its treatment), such as nausea and vomiting, diarrhoea, and failure to absorb food that is eaten, can all contribute to weight loss.

Prolonged loss of appetite (anorexia) leads to wasting which is known as cachexia. The symptoms of this condition, which is common in advanced cancer, are:

● Increasing emaciation.
● Generalized and progressive weakness.
● Loss of appetite—the thought or smell of food usually revolts the patient.
● Changes in the body's hormones.

The condition is difficult to treat because a vicious circle develops: the more you lose weight the less you want to eat. Relatives become concerned and often press patients to eat a normal meal in order to make them 'stronger' but this is impossible.It is better to eat small meals of anything you may fancy. In addition many patients have poor or altered taste so that even if you feel hungry you may be dissuaded by the smell of food. Food that looks good but which does not have a strong smell may be more acceptable. 'Tasty' foods are usually preferred to bland foods.

Alcohol or 'tonics' before meals may help improve appetite but the only generally successful treatment is steroids. Prednisone tablets will increase appetite and often improve mood and make patients generally feel better. Food supplements containing protein and with a high calorie content may also be useful. They can be obtained in various flavours, though many patients find them tasteless. The names of some commercial preparations include:

Build-up
Caloreen
Casilan
Clinifeed
Hycal

Patients who are likely to respond to anticancer treatment may be given infusions of special high calorie and protein mixtures into a vein. This is known as intravenous hyperalimentation and it is used to build up a patient who is weak or ill. It must be done in hospital and a fine plastic catheter (tube) is usually put into a vein in the neck. It is the surest way of feeding up a patient, but is only justified if the patient's cancer is being treated, as it is complicated. Alternatively, a fine plastic tube may be passed through the nose and into the patient's stomach; feeds are injected through the tube.

DRY MOUTH

This is a common symptom that is often due to a combination of factors. The commonest of these are:

- Certain drugs, especially pain-killers, antidepressants, sedatives, and antisickness drugs.
- Radiotherapy to the neck or jaws.
- Decreased body fluids (dehydration).
- Poor appetite.
- Mouth breathing.

Sometimes treatment that is causing the dry mouth can be stopped, but usually it is only possible to try to increase the patient's saliva. Patients can do this by sucking acid sweets (such as lemon drops) or chewing gum. If the problem is severe, artificial saliva can be prescribed and dehydration reversed by replacing lost fluids.

SORE MOUTH

This may also be due to a variety of causes:

- Fungus infections (monilia, commonly known as thrush).
- Drug reactions (Appendix A and Chapter 12).
- Aphthous ulcers.
- Vitamin deficiencies.
- Bacterial infections.
- Cold sores (herpes simplex).

If your normal immunity is reduced you may be prone to a fungal infection called monilia (thrush). Steroids, antibiotics, and anticancer drugs all increase the risk of this infection and as all three types of drugs are used in cancer patients it is not surprising that monilia mouth infections are common.

Careful cleansing of the mouth is, therefore, very important in order to avoid or reduce the problem. Teeth should be cleaned 3–4 times a day with a soft toothbrush and at times of high risk dentures should be removed except for meals. Non-alcohol-containing mouthwashes should be used 3–4 times a day (see page 87). Corsodyl, oraldene and betadine mouthwashes are commercial preparations that are available. Diflam oral rinse is an anaesthetic mouthwash which is useful for reducing discomfort.

If a fungal infection does develop then antifungal lozenges and mouthwashes should be used. Available treatments (brand name in brackets) used include:

(1) Amphoteracin (Fungilin) lozenges, which should be dissolved slowly in the mouth or taken in suspension which is used as a mouthwash then swallowed. Both should be used at least 4 times a day.
(2) Miconazole (Daktarin) gel which is used to rinse the mouth at least 4 times a day.

(3) Nystatin (Nystatin) suspension used to rinse the mouth at least 4 times a day.

(4) Ketoconazole (Nizoral) is a new drug which is absorbed into the body.

Aphthous ulcers are small painful ulcers that develop on the gums and inside the lips. They can occur in anyone at any time but are more common at times of stress or illness. Hydrocortisone lozenges (Corlan) can be useful if they are held in the mouth against the ulcer. Carbenoxolene (Bioral gel), and Bonjella can also be applied to an ulcer to deaden pain.

Only rarely do vitamins improve a sore mouth, but if there is a specific vitamin deficiency they will be helpful. Anticancer drugs may damage the lining (mucosa) of the mouth and temporary soreness and ulceration are common. Good hygiene is important and if no bacterial or fungal infection develops this will recover after 4–7 days. If a sore mouth is caused by the drug methotrexate (see Appendix A) folinic acid mouthwashes help healing.

DIFFICULTY IN SWALLOWING

If there is narrowing of the oesophagus (gullet) or if a tumour presses on the oesophagus this will cause difficulty in swallowing (known as dysphagia). Though some cancers can respond quickly to chemotherapy or radiotherapy, the ones that commonly cause difficulty in swallowing do not. An operation to insert a special tube through the tumour is often very helpful (page 109) allowing the patient to eat normally.

Not all patients with difficulty in swallowing have tumour in or pressing on the gullet and it is important to find out the cause. Sometimes fungal infections of the mouth (candida) spread down the oesophagus and cause painful difficulty in swallowing.

OBSTRUCTION OF THE BOWEL
(INTESTINAL OBSTRUCTION)

Obstruction or blockage of the bowel is most common in cancers of the large bowel and ovary. It usually starts slowly with occasional episodes of colicky pain in the abdomen. A colicky pain is one that comes and goes, like the pain we may get if we eat too many green apples. The pain is often accompanied by loud bowel sounds, swelling of the abdomen and sometimes diarrhoea. The symptoms of complete bowel obstruction are:

- Colicky abdominal pain.
- Nausea.
- Then vomiting.
- Constipation which becomes so complete that even wind is not passed.
- Waves of muscular contractions in the bowel that may occasionally be visible through the wall of the abdomen.

If you have these symptoms see a doctor immediately; if there is complete bowel obstruction you will probably need to be treated in hospital. Initially the bowel is rested by stopping food and fluids; these are given by an intravenous infusion (drip) into the vein. If nausea or vomiting is severe, a tube (nasogastric tube) is passed through the nose into the stomach and excess fluids sucked off. This is uncomfortable but rapidly relieves any nausea. In many cases the obstruction will settle with this simple treatment. If it does not surgery may be considered. Such operations are usually confined to patients with a cancer of the large bowel but often mean that a colostomy (pages 111 and 291) is necessary. If the cancer cannot be operated on then radiotherapy (page 71) or chemotherapy (page 80) can occasionally be helpful. Even if these treatments are not useful, intravenous fluids (drip), and suction of the stomach contents will often 'settle' the blockage down and, when used together with pain-killers and antisickness drugs, can remove the unpleasant symptoms.

If the cancer is very advanced, operations, nasogastric tubes, and infusions may not be necessary as drugs can provide relief without the need for any unpleasant or distressing treatment. The care of intestinal obstruction depends entirely on the extent of the tumour.

- If the patient is not known to have cancer an operation will be required to make the diagnosis, and this may be curative if there is only a localized bowel cancer.
- Patients with recurrent or progressive disease. If the patient

has bowel cancer affecting one part of the bowel only, an operation can provide good relief but is rarely curative. In the case of recurrent ovarian cancer operations are rarely helpful and other treatments should generally be considered.

- For some patients there will be no treatment that can control the tumour, but it is important to remember that treatment can be used to help the symptoms.

Remember abdominal pains, nausea, and bowel upsets are common in patients with cancer and are usually *not* due to an obstruction. However, if you have the symptoms mentioned above, seek medical advice early.

COLLECTION OF FLUID IN THE ABDOMEN (ASCITES)

Sometimes a tumour causes fluid to accumulate in the abdominal cavity and this can lead to uncomfortable swelling and difficulty in breathing just like that in pregnancy. The discomfort can be eased quickly by aspirating (drawing off) the fluid. A narrow plastic tube (catheter) is inserted through the skin of the abdomen (after an injection of local anaesthetic) and the fluid is sucked up into a syringe or a suction bottle. This may take several hours, is usually not too painful and dramatically relieves the symptoms. The procedure is usually done in hospital.

Sometimes a drug, usually bleomycin (Appendix A), is injected through the tube to try to prevent the fluid returning. If possible, specific anticancer treatment, radiotherapy, or chemotherapy should also be used to stop reaccumulation of the ascites.

INCREASED CALCIUM IN THE BLOOD (HYPERCALCAEMIA)

Calcium is normally held in bones and teeth, but in some cancers large amounts are released into the blood. When this happens the following effects are seen:

- Constipation.
- Nausea and vomiting.
- Loss of appetite.
- Drowsiness and confusion.

- Weakness.

Immediate treatment is large quantities of fluid, given by an intravenous infusion (drip). If this does not reduce the high level of calcium, steroids or other drugs can be used to reduce the calcium level.

It is also important to try to plan therapy to shrink the cancer itself. The only sure way to get rid of the symptoms of hypercalcaemia is to get rid of the cause of the raised calcium—the cancer itself.

Unless a patient is really very ill, admission to hospital for a short period is advisable if hypercalcaemia develops. The use of infusions and drugs will get rid of the symptoms and, if possible, anticancer treatment can then be planned.

SHORTNESS OF BREATH

Shortness of breath, often with a cough, is not uncommon in advanced cancer. There are many possible causes, some unrelated to cancer, but the commonest are:

- Tumour in the lung.
- Development of a collection of fluid in the chest (a pleural effusion).
- Scarring of the lungs after radiation or chemotherapy.
- Severe anaemia.
- Infection in the lung.

If there is tumour in the lung, specific anticancer therapy will, if possible, be used. When a pleural effusion develops, the shortness of breath it causes can be improved by draining off the fluid (pleural aspiration). This may be done in two ways:

(1) If the fluid has not previously been troublesome, then a thin needle is pushed through the chest wall (between the ribs) into the fluid (page 56). The fluid is sucked out using a syringe or suction bottle and the needle is then taken out. It is done after an injection of a local anaesthetic and takes about half an hour.
(2) If the fluid keeps returning, then a small operation is performed to put a plastic tube (catheter) into the chest. This is done under local anaesthetic and only takes a few minutes.

The plastic catheter is then connected to a bottle with water in it—this stops air getting back into the chest—and the fluid in the chest is slowly sucked out until none is left. A drug is then injected through the tube into the chest in an attempt to stop the fluid coming back. This type of treatment is successful in over half of the cases and is well worth trying. Patients will be in hospital for about 2–3 days. The tube may be mildly uncomfortable and can interfere with sleep whilst it is in the chest, but it is removed once the fluid has been taken away and the injection given. Some drugs used for the injection can cause pain or fever.

Inflammation of the lungs may start several months after radiation has been given to the chest. It is often accompanied by a cough and feeling of being generally unwell. Steroids quickly relieve the inflammation and symptoms. The dose of steroids (usually prednisone tablets) must be reduced very gradually as the inflammation will return if they are stopped suddenly. Shortness of breath, developing some years after radiotherapy, which is caused by radiation scarring (fibrosis) is more difficult to treat and cannot be reversed.

Severe anaemia is easily treated with a blood transfusion and patients often feel much better afterwards. Most patients are not short of iron and iron tablets are usually not helpful.

Infections are common (page 88) and require treatment with antibiotics, but viruses or any other unusual infections can be difficult to treat.

COUGH

If a cough is caused by a specific problem that can be treated (for instance, bronchitis treated with an antibiotic) this is clearly the treatment of choice. If such treatment is not available 'cough mixtures' (antitussives) are needed. These act locally in the lungs or centrally in the brain.

Local action

(1) Expectorants. Drugs that stimulate the cough and make it more effective by increasing the lungs' secretions. They may or may not help.

(2) Mucolytics. Drugs that reduce the stickiness of the lung secretions. The commonest is bromhexine (Bisolvon is the trade name). One or two tablets can be taken 3 times a day and there is a liquid form.

(3) Decongestants. There are a great number of these, often combining a decongestant (usually ephedrine) with an antihistamine and codeine. Commonly used drugs include Actifed compound lintus and phensedyl cough linctus and they often seem to help patients.

Central action

The commonest drugs, in increasing strength, are:

(1) Codeine linctus.
(2) Pholcodeine linctus.
(3) Methadone linctus.
(4) Diamorphine linctus.

They all act as cough suppressants.

It is often best to combine two drugs acting in different ways, e.g. a mucolytic (bromhexine) and codeine linctus.

URINARY INCONTINENCE

This is rather a common and distressing symptom in severely ill patients and there are several reasons why it happens.

- Urinary infections. These are common and cause increased frequency of urination and pain on passing urine as well as occasional incontinence. Treatment is with an antibiotic.
- Cancer irritating or pressing on the bladder can cause increased frequency of passing urine and occasionally incontinence. Treatment is designed to shrink the tumour (surgery, radiotherapy, or chemotherapy). Treatment with radiation to the bladder can cause scarring and shrinkage and the drugs, cyclophosphamide and ifosphamide, can cause irradiation of the bladder (Appendix A).
- Interference with nerves to the bladder. Occasionally cancer can press on the spinal cord and interfere with the way the bladder functions. This is usually accompanied with weakness of the legs and loss or altered sensation in the lower half of

the body. *Immediate* radiotherapy or surgery to remove the pressure on the spinal cord should always be arranged in all but the most ill patients. If this condition is not treated urgently paralysis of the legs and permanent incontinence will develop. Anyone with weakness of their legs, loss or change of sensation, or unexplained incontinence should get the advice of their doctor quickly.

- Passing increased quantities of urine (polyuria). This is often due to diabetes, which is treated in the usual way. Kidney failure can also cause this problem, its treatment will depend on the cause.

Catheterization

If incontinence cannot be controlled easily, a thin tube (catheter) is passed into the bladder. This should be done in a sterile manner and the catheter is kept in place by a small balloon which is inflated when the catheter is in the bladder; this is painless. If a catheter is needed over a long period then it should be changed regularly (about once a month) and each change of catheter covered by two days' antibiotics to prevent the introduction of bacteria into the bladder.

The use of a catheter is extremely important if there is persistent incontinence. It is very important to avoid leakage of urine as this may result in infection, sores and ulcers, making life miserable. Often, quite wrongly, catheterization is unnecessarily delayed. Nobody wants a catheter, but it can make life bearable if incontinence is uncontrolled.

URINARY RETENTION (THE INABILITY TO PASS URINE)

This is less common but usually requires catheterization until the cause can be taken away (for example an operation for an enlarged prostate).

LACK OF SLEEP (INSOMNIA)

Many patients who are severely ill suffer from insomnia because of pain, anxiety, frequency of urination, and shortness of breath. If lack of sleep is due to depression then specific treatment is needed. Pain should be treated (page 264) with adequate, regular doses of pain-killers. If sedatives are needed to help a patient to sleep, the best drugs are those falling into a group called benzodiazepins. The best known of these is diazepam (Valium is the trade name) and another, nitrazepam (Mogadon) is also commonly used. The dose is 5–10 mg taken at night. Elderly patients who become confused by these drugs may be better off with chloral (trade name—Welldorm) or chlormethiazole (Hemineverin). Temazepam is a useful drug as its breakdown products are not active. For those who are awakened by severe sweating (common in some types of cancer) indomethacin (Indocid) tablets can be helpful.

DEPRESSION

Most people with cancer will suffer some degree of depression. It is a normal response to learning of serious illness and is common during treatment. This 'reactive' depression often responds best to sympathetic discussion, but sometimes people become emotionally exhausted by months of worry and gradually become apathetic; it is this apathy that can quickly turn to real depression. Depression removes the will to recover and needs urgent treatment.

Modern antidepressant tablets, given as a single dose at night—the commonest are called tricyclics—can do much to help lift mood and allows an opportunity for discussion with a skilled therapist or doctor. Treatment for pain or any worrying symptom must not be ignored as this may do much to relieve depression. Depression is often coupled with anxiety and this is discussed below.

ANXIETY

Anxiety is characterized by a collection of unpleasant nervous symptoms: it is the body's response to excess stress and tension. Once this is seen as the problem, it is important to realize that these feelings are of no medical significance, though they are very bewildering and distressing. It may be set off by:

- Worries about curability.
- Fear of treatment.

- Fear of being in hospital.
- Fear of future symptoms.
- Financial worries.
- Worries about outpatient visits.
- Worries about spouse and children.
- Spiritual worries.

Apart from the constant feelings of tension, other physical symptoms occur in 'attacks'—panic spasms, palpitations, chest pain, giddiness, nausea, trembling spells, inability to take a deep breath, difficulty in swallowing, as well as depression and sleeplessness.

It is helpful if your doctor can take time to listen to your fears; this is often more useful than drugs. Drugs (usually diazepam) may be useful initially to help settle the symptoms, but regular discussions will keep problems in perspective and often eventually helps to calm fears. A clear explanation of the symptoms themselves and the fact that the cause is emotional rather than physical is important to anyone suffering from anxiety. This explanation can itself help the patient to find peace of mind. Emotional problems are more upsetting than physical distress for relatives, but can often be helped by sympathetic care.

RESTLESSNESS AND CONFUSION

It is very upsetting when a close relative eventually fails to recognize anyone, becomes disorientated, noisy, and restless. Sometimes it is caused by drugs and a dose adjustment will help, but often the cause is not easy to find. Confused patients are greatly helped by seeing familiar faces and being (if possible) in their own surroundings. Restlessness or aggressive confusion can be helped by drugs such as chlorpromazine.

CARE OF ULCERATING CANCERS

A minority of cancers grow in the skin and become ulcerated. This is particularly distressing as the cancer is now visible or may even smell. If possible, treatment with radiotherapy, or chemotherapy should be used to reduce the tumour. It is most common in cancer of the breast and disfigurement of this sort is particularly difficult for women—especially a scrupulously clean woman to bear. Often patients isolate themselves and are distressed thinking that they smell.

- If there is infection, a seven-day course of a broad-spectrum antibiotic is given. This reduces infection and any unpleasant smell.
- The ulcerated area should be cleaned often, 2 or 3 times a day. Eusol diluted half and half with water is very helpful, though this may be uncomfortable in sensitive areas. Betadine and Hibitane (trade names) are alternative antiseptics that do not sting. If the area is ulcerated and wet then eusol (50 per cent) with paraffin (50 per cent) can be applied to the area using gauze soaked in the solution. If the area is dry it can be cleaned with a salt solution (saline) and a dry dressing applied. Gentian violet is often very effective for drying moist ulcers.
- If there is bleeding from the ulcer (especially from where it sticks to a dressing) a special non-adhesive dressing should be used.

Sometimes radiotherapy can be useful. There is seldom need to fear a sudden haemorrhage, as many patients do. With careful dressing and care, often by a visiting nurse, the problems of a large ulcerated area can be minimized.

CHAPTER 51

Talking about cancer

Cancer is the disease people are most frightened about. It is a subject fraught with myth, mystery, and most of all silence. It is usually assumed that all cancers are painful and fatal; a disease for which there is 'no cure' and 'no hope'. However, there has been much progress in the control of cancer, and this is not widely understood.

There is a gradual awareness amongst those looking after cancer patients, led by cancer sufferers, that an honest approach to the situation is the most sensible and right policy and we have assumed that anyone wishing to read this book will be looking for the truth, however sad it may sometimes seem.

After a cancer has been found a decision must be made whether the patient should be told. In the past doctors have talked around the diagnosis using cryptic words such as 'ulcers', 'cysts', 'lesions'; but recently it has become more usual to discuss the diagnosis openly with the patient. Most people seem to find it easier to deal with the disease and its treatment if they understand exactly what is going on. For many it is just the confirmation of what they had strongly suspected. In situations where the patient is not told but close family are given the diagnosis, this can be very destructive: the patient becomes isolated and the family lie to maintain the fiction. Usually the patient is aware of the cancer, but cannot discuss it with husband or wife for fear of causing distress, whilst the spouse knows too but is also frightened of talking about it. This causes imaginable tension.

For most of us, a simple knowledge of the disease and its treatment is helpful and we want any questions answered with honesty tempered with sensitivity. This book should answer some questions, but is only intended as a back-up to your discussion with those looking after you; it cannot be stressed too strongly that a good relationship with those caring for you is very important. Try to find someone with whom you can easily discuss your treatment, fears and worries, be it the family doctor, a nurse, or a good friend. Discussions with medical staff, including those about tests, treatment, and prognosis and what it means for you should proceed at a pace that you can handle comfortably. If you lead the discussion the correct pace is assured. A good proportion of this book deals with how and why the patient is treated; but every hospital has its own way of doing things, and it is useful to ask about the treatment and investigations that are being planned for you. Some hospitals prepare a short leaflet outlining the treatment and its side-effects; ask if you can have one.

Surprisingly little research has been done into emotional reactions to cancer, even though difficulties caused by poor communication, treatment, pain, and changes in role or life style are very common. These problems usually parallel three different stages of the disease (remember many patients do **not** have advancing disease). The initial phase is the time cancer is detected and diagnosed. An intermediate phase is when treatent is under way, but the outcome for success or failure is uncertain. For some there is an advancing phase when treatment has failed to control the tumour, and death must be faced.

DETECTION

The discovery of a strange and worrying lump or persistent symptom that doesn't go away on its own, is often as shocking as learning for the first that it it is indeed cancer. The apparent gravity of the diagnosis may be compounded by the doctor's silence, his uncomfortable 'small talk', serious manner, or vain reassurance. We are often afraid to ask what is wrong, and so a conspiracy of silence develops.

Next follows a period of waiting for the outcome of exhaustive tests and biopsies which follow the initial examination. This is a very trying time; if you want to know about the tests, ask.

WHEN CANCER IS DIAGNOSED

When the diagnosis has been made and confirmed an open and friendly talk with everyone concerned is often valuable. It clears the air and opens the path for questions and frank discussion of fears and feelings; but all too often this does not happen, with the result that the patient becomes visibly withdrawn and depressed or is tearful and family and friends try to ignore what is happening and a tense situation builds up. Some people are very open and composed about their illness and are keen to discuss it, but again some find such free expression of a 'taboo' subject uncomfortable. Perhaps it is most sensible to find a wise counsellor, preferably a doctor or any experienced friend, who can view problems from a detached point of view. Though a platitude, 'a trouble shared is a trouble halved' is often very true for the cancer patient.

Coping with death

Coming to terms with dying is very difficult for anyone to imagine. Anger, fear and bitterness at the situation a common reaction.

It seems, to the patient, that those who care little for life live to an old age, whilst those who revel in its challenges are stricken with illness prematurely. Anger follows, caused by the threat of death, and is then followed by a painful sense of bitterness which is often not recognized by others.

In their effort to help the patient repress unpleasant emotions and sometimes to defend themselves against anxiety, others make it hard for the patient to express feelings. Communication is further hampered by the patient's own guilt over the anger he feels and depression follows and family and friends, taking their cue from the patient, leave him alone or become anxious or irritated—and a communication stalemate results. Often visitors are tense and ill-at-ease and the patient ends up making cheery conversation about everything but their real feelings. Feelings of bitterness are, therefore, not readily got rid of. Sadness, tears, and helplessness are easily understood and result in empathy; bitterness does not and patients quickly learn this and avoid expressing it.

Remember that:

- Denial and anger often need to be expressed.
- Self-pity in small doses helps a lot—so grumble.
- Your feelings are respectable, so don't feel guilty.

- Discussion of feelings is often best *not* done with relatives who are too involved.
- It is not wicked to hate doctors, family or God.
- Vent your feelings—'kicking the cat' is healthy.
- Try to be realistic. The dying have a great freedom—nothing more can happen to you so do what you want. You can become a great risk-taker; the rest of us are too afraid of risks.
- Guilt should be assuaged.

CONTINUING PROBLEMS

- No matter how great your optimism there is often a nagging awareness that cancer *might* return. Although with time this lessens, it is nontheless there. No-one can be completely reassured and sometimes this eventually makes family and friends angry. Patients having a check-up years after their cancer was treated often feel anxious and unwell for several days before seeing their doctor; no-one emerges from the experience as if it had never happened, like all bad experiences.
- Treatment, especially surgery, may disfigure and this is especially important with certain operations such as mastectomy. For weeks after such an operation you may find it difficult to look at the scar. Patients often hate how they look and feel depressed and over-react to any new loss. Dressing and undressing are a painful reminder of the loss and wearing some clothes becomes unthinkable, despite assurance that a prosthesis would make you look normal.
- Pain is depressing, frightening and tiring, and is very difficult to describe. Because of this it is important to ensure that every effort is made to control any pain (page 264).
- Open communication cannot resolve all the problems but for most it certainly helps. Empathetic support from all concerned makes the unbearable possible to bear, and many who think that they will never cope often show great strength and resilience which surprises even themselves.

DYING

Most of this book is concerned with the active treatment of cancer and the enormous advances that have occurred in the past 10–20 years. Unfortunately some patients die from their tumour. If you have been told that nothing more can be done, this is seldom if ever true.

Methods for controlling symptoms (Chapter 50) continue to get better and 'active' treatment to improve your quality of life become as important as earlier treatments that attempted 'cure'. Unfortunately, all too often the transition from treatment to cure cancer to treatment for symptoms only is made arbitrarily and suddenly. It has been said that the dying (or terminal) phase of a disease can be defined as beginning at the moment the doctor says, 'Nothing more can be done', and then withdraws from the patient. What he really means is that there is nothing more surgically to be done (if he is a surgeon) or no radiotherapy or chemotherapy will help (if he is a radiotherapist). The same is true for all other specialists.

Because communication has often been poor earlier in the disease you may find it difficult to become involved in decisions regarding further therapy. A rational decision is very difficult and you should never be asked to make decisions by yourself. It is the physician's job to explore the possibilities and then to arrive at a conclusion in discussion with you and often your family. Occasionally two treatments will have equal merit. We all like to be involved with our own destiny and nothing generates a better relationship between patient and doctor.

If a decision is made to stop 'curative' treatment it is imperative that you do not feel that you are being abandoned. Doctors often (because of their impotence and sense of failure) feel threatened by a dying patient and respond by gradually ignoring them, but this is when you need the greatest time and skill from your doctor. The increasing number of hospices (also called continuing care units) emphasizes the general lack of these skills that still exist. Continuing care units are not special places for the dying; they are as the name implies, units concerned with improving the quality of life of the cancer patient. They have expertise in the treatment of symptoms and relief of physical and mental distress that allows the patient to concentrate on living as full a life as possible. The aim of most hospices is to get patients home to their family and friends and most have a team of specialist doctors and nurses who will support the patient at home in any way they can. The most common reaction of patients to hospices is what happy places they are!

The patient

If you have had a surgical treatment that caused loss of part of your body you are likely to need adequate time to get over or mourn this loss. If your family, friends and doctor are made uncomfortable by this, you could need professional counselling. The longer this process of adjustment is delayed the greater is the likelihood of depression. This process takes time, but surprisingly patients adjust to loss much more effectively than do most relatives.

Similar reactions occur with radiotherapy and chemotherapy and do not be surprised by the feelings of depression, anger (often irritational anger or irritability), bitterness, sadness, and deep disappointment which will occur; they are quite normal reactions to all that is happening. Patients often prefer to be with close relatives and friends during this time to obtain mutual support.

Family and friends

To the family and close friends a cancer patient is someone who is probably suffering physical and mental pain. You are shocked and feel helpless, not knowing what to say or how to express the things you want to say. You may suddenly be faced with the possibility of death, loss of a loved one, and wonder how to prepare for this without showing the patient what you dread to admit to yourself. Whilst you are feeling these things the patient struggles with how he has let you down and frantically wishes he could wave a magic wand to change the reality of these terrible events. Patients wonder if family and friends will be able to stay with them through all this, but cannot ask for fear that they won't be understood or will upset their relatives by fearfulness and excessive dependency. Most patients need to be 'forgiven' for their illness; any severe illness places added burdens on those around the patient and they are aware of this. They also need to be reassured that their cancer is not a punishment for past misdeeds.

Advice to helpers

A relative, friend, or doctor who wants to help a patient must let them know that they are not going to desert them and that they are trying to understand some of the struggles the patient is experiencing. Someone to whom they can talk as little or as much as they want without embarrassment is often the best support. Patience and an ability to *listen* rather than to give advice is usually best. Tell the patient of your optimism and hope (if this is appropriate) but be realistic, never maudlin or pessimistic. Go with the patient if you can, to check-ups, radiotherapy, chemotherapy, or any hospital visits. Show pleasure with any progress but do not try to push the patient back to health. Daily expressions of 'you do look better today' when the patient is getting worse are stupid and can only cause frustration, anger, and resentment. It is hard to resist the temptation, but don't do it. Be aware that ups and downs and periods of irritability, depression and dependency are common. This is difficult for friends and relatives and you must be able to let off steam with others and may need advice from your family doctor or friends.

Families and friends must, above all, remember that the patient needs to mourn. You must allow the patient time to grieve, accepting that it is a normal, healthy process which he must pass painfully through in order to get successfully over loss and to resolve depression. As mentioned before patients do it much better than relatives—even if their emotional reactions may appear more dramatic.

In the hospital

Communication with doctors is particularly difficult and most patients feel more comfortable with and talk more openly to nurses. Doctors are too powerful, they can give 'good' or 'bad' news, for the relationship to be easy. In addition the doctor plays out his role together with the patient and this traditional role puts obligations, which may suppress open discussion, on both. If there is hope, then it is best that it is given quickly and clearly to the patient. Most patients feel too frightened to ask threatening questions and use many devices, such as telling themselves, 'I'll wait till I'm stronger', to avoid asking. It is easy for a doctor to discourage questions by his attitude; this may be excessively reassuring or defensive. Some doctors may even seem to criticize a lack of questions but it is best for the patient to make the pace, they should be given every opportunity to question but never have unwanted information forced on them. The doctor–patient relationship is complicated by each other's perception of the cancer and their response on it. The patient may in some way sense that they have disappointed or failed their doctor by having such an onerous disease or by failing treatment. They may feel that the physician would rather not see them because there is no 'cure' and this is compounded by the doctor's feeling of inadequacy and failure in the face of a difficult or even insoluble problem.

Patients with advancing cancer, in addition to sympathetic and skilled psychological support, need expert treatment to control symptoms. Some of the methods of treatment used are described in Chapter 50 and it is very important that care is taken to ensure that every measure is used to control physical problems. This may frequently be done by hospital doctors working together with the patient's GP but sometimes it is useful for the patient to have the help of a team of doctors or nurses from a continuing care centre.

CHAPTER 52

Ostomies: colostomies, ileostomies and urinary diversions

An ostomy is a surgical operation to make a new pathway for the discharge of the body's wastes; the opening on to the surface of skin is known as a stoma. These operations are done for a number of diseases of the bowel and urinary tract including cancer.

When the new opening is formed from the colon the stoma is called a colostomy and when it is formed from the ileum (part of the small bowel) the stoma is known as an ileostomy. Both these stomas discharge faeces, but the one chosen will depend on where the cancer is.

In cancer of the bladder it may be necessary to remove totally the bladder and the ureters (tubes that connect the kidneys and bladder) may be brought directly up to the skin or may be connected to the ileum (part of the small bowel) which is brought up to the skin as a stoma (this is called an ileal conduit).

After an ostomy operation a patient loses voluntary control over the discharge of the wastes concerned and has to wear a special appliance for the collection of this waste. Despite this, there is no reason why a patient with a stoma should not live a perfectly normal life: family, social, business, and sporting. However, adjustment is difficult and patients need help in learning to live with their ostomy. Some find it difficult to manage the appliance, but even if this is no problem they may find it impossible to resume a normal social life. Help from special stoma nurses and ostomy associations is available even before an operation is done and it is well worth patients contacting local associations. Members of these groups usually have an ostomy themselves and can give practical help and encouragement from their own experience. Although many colostomies are permanent, some may be temporary and these are usually done when an operation has relieved a bowel obstruction. A temporary colostomy may be removed after several months and the normal bowel joined together again.

COLOSTOMIES

A colostomy may be a *sigmoid, descending, tranverse* or *ascending* colostomy depending on which part of the colon is used to make the stoma (Figure 42). If properly cared for and fitted the appliance can be completely odourless and invisible to others.

Descending and sigmoid colostomies

This is usually a permanent operation and is most commonly done when it is impossible to remove a cancer that is low down in the bowel without causing incontinence. The remaining part of the colon still absorbs water and because of this semi-solid stool will probably be formed.

Some patients may eventually have motions at more or less regular times during the day and can manage without a bag for part of the day (a stoma cap is adequate). Irrigation or enemas can be used to regulate the colostomy to prevent 'unscheduled' movements though this should only be done on a doctor's advice.

Transverse colostomy

This is often a temporary colostomy. The nature of discharge is unpredictable though it is usually semi-liquid and a stoma appliance is usually worn continuously. As the discharge contains digestive enzymes the appliance used must protect the skin around the stoma and special seals are used.

Ascending colon

The discharge is liquid and flows almost continuously. Because it contains digestive enzymes protection of the skin around the stoma is important. It is usually looked after in the same way as an ileostomy (see below) and a special seal is needed around the stoma.

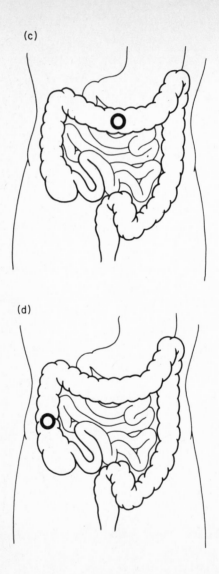

Figure 42 Diagrammatic representation of the large bowel showing the different positions where a stoma may be placed. (a) sigmoid colostomy, (b) descending colostomy, (c) transverse colostomy, (d) ascending colostomy

(a)

(b)

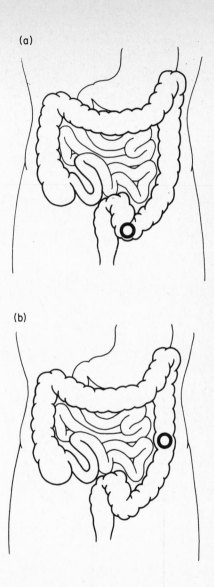

Figure 42 (*contd*)

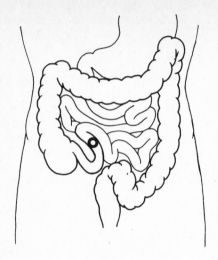

Figure 43 Diagrammatic representation of the position of an ileostomy stoma

ILEOSTOMY

This ostomy is made using the ileum, the part of the small intestine farthest from the stomach (Figure 43). An ileostomy is usually performed using the last part of the ileum just before the colon and is often done when the whole of the colon and rectum is removed in an operation designed to prevent cancer (page 5).

As there is no longer a colon to absorb water and form solid stools the ileostomy discharges liquid which flows almost continuously. This contains digestive enzymes and the ileostomy stoma is made to protrude up to an inch into the appliance so that the skin is protected. This is very important because the enzymes will digest the skin and cause the appliance to leak which in turn worsens the problem.

After operations requiring an ileostomy the aim must be total rehabilitation. Skin protection is basic and a properly fitted appliance is essential. An ideal appliance should be simple to put on, provide a leak-proof seal, and be odourless. Because they change in size and shape the stoma should be re-measured periodically and the appliance changed as required.

ILEAL CONDUIT

This operation is so-termed because the surgeon converts a segment of the ileum (about 15 cm) into a pipe, or conduit, for urinary drainage. The ureters are disconnected from the bladder (which is usually removed) and are joined to one end of the ileum, the other end of the ileum being brought through the abdominal wall to form a stoma. The segment of ileum removed from the small intestine survives on its own blood supply and the rest of the bowel is rejoined and continues to work normally.

There is no 'voluntary' control of the stoma which discharges a drop of urine every 10–20 seconds. A urostomy bag is worn over the stoma and should be leak-proof, easily fitted, odourless, and have the facility for night drainage.

Details on the use of ostomy appliances can be obtained from the various associations and groups included in Appendix C. Patients with an ostomy can, in the United Kingdom, apply for a certificate of exemption from prescription charges for equipment available under the National Health Service.

CHAPTER 53

Understanding the way hospitals work

This chapter describes briefly how you, as a patient, will be cared for, once a suspicious symptom has been noticed. After you have decided to seek advice, it tells you about the role of the medical staff you will meet along the way.

When a strange lump, or odd bleeding, or a persistent cough refuses to go away, the first step is to make an appointment to see your GP. He will make a thorough examination, and if he thinks the problem needs further investigation he will write a letter to a hospital doctor, usually a surgeon, describing his findings, and asking him to see you. If he feels the problem is urgent he will say so, and the waiting time should not be very long.

You will receive a letter from the appointments department at your nearest General Hospital, telling you when and where to attend, and the name of the consultant surgeon you will expect to see. On the day, when you reach the hospital, one of the clerical staff will ask you for various details (name, address, date of birth) and these will be entered in your file of notes. Each file has its own number, so it can be traced easily, and produced at your appointments.

Out-patient departments are notoriously unpunctual, and you may have to wait a while to be seen; so it is advisable to allow yourself plenty of time off, if you have a job. Before seeing the doctor, a nurse will weigh you, and ask for a urine specimen.

When you go in to see the surgeon, he will take a full history, give you a detailed examination, and then discuss what he thinks is wrong. At this point, he will, if necessary, arrange special tests or a 'biopsy'. A biopsy, or the taking away of a small piece of tissue for microscopic examination, is often a minor procedure, and may well be done on a day-case basis. He may also send you along for a chest X-ray, and some routine blood tests. If you wish to, feel free to ask how and why the tests are being done—most hospitals will try to be helpful.

The results of the biopsy will confirm the diagnosis, and if cancer cells are found you will be contacted immediately, and admission to hospital arranged for surgery, or an out-patient appointment for other treatment (chemotherapy or radio-therapy). This will be discussed with you by the consultant or ward medical staff. If you are to be admitted, go straight to the ward indicated on your admissions slip and the ward clerk will check through your details.

The consultant or senior registrar will come and see you and go through a 'plan of action' for your particular cancer. This may involve surgery, chemotherapy, radiotherapy—one, or maybe all three. A radiotherapist will come and tell you about any radiation treatment, and a medical oncologist about drug treatment. When you return home, you will be given a 'follow up' appointment to be seen by your doctor in the out-patient department to make sure that you are feeling well, and to continue any drug, or other treatment you may need. The hospital doctors looking after you will write to your GP so that he knows all the details of your cancer and its treatment. When treatment has finished you will be given further 'follow up' appointments at regular intervals, whose frequency will decrease the longer you remain disease-free.

If problems do crop up between appointments go back and see your GP. He will know all about your illness, and put you in touch with the hospital, so that you can be seen again quickly. If you want to know more about your illness and its treatment, ask the doctors and nurses looking after you—most are only too happy to answer your questions.

THE MEDICAL STAFF

Consultant Physician or Surgeon

He is the boss, and is in charge of a team of doctors called 'a firm'. It is his name that appears on your bed-card, and your care is ultimately his responsibility. In an academic unit, where there are medical students, the consultant may be known by the title 'Professor'.

Senior Registrar

He is second in command, and will be extremely well qualified in his field. He is more obviously available than the consultant, and will spend more time on the ward.

Registrar

He is younger and more junior than the Senior Registrar, but none the less, well qualified. He keeps an eye on the housemen, and will be present on ward rounds to check the day-to-day progress of each patient.

House Surgeon or House Physician

He is quite recently qualified, and looks after the day-to-day running of the ward. He works long hours and will spend some nights living in the hospital when the firm is on call. He will be most available for you, or your relatives, to talk over any worries or problems, on a day-to-day basis.

Medical students

If you are in a teaching hospital, you will encounter medical students. They are training to become doctors, and you may be asked whether you mind being examined by them for teaching purposes, either on the wards, or in the clinic. You can always say no, if you don't want this.

Anaesthetist

He is the doctor who puts you to sleep and keeps an eye on your breathing during an operation. You will possibly first encounter him the day before an operation when he checks that you are fit for an anaesthetic.

THE NURSING STAFF

Sister

She is an experienced state registered nurse (SRN), and she is in charge of the ward or department. Its smooth running is her responsibility, and traditionally she wears a navy blue uniform.

Staff Nurse

She is a state registered nurse, who has passed her final examinations, and will be highly qualified and competent. It is usually possible to identify an SRN by her plain dark belt and silver buckle.

State enrolled nurse

A state enrolled nurse or SEN will wear a different coloured uniform from a sister or a staff nurse. Her training is shorter than that of an SRN and she will be more concerned with practical work on the ward.

Also on the ward, will be student nurses at various stages of training and auxiliary nurses who are not formally trained at all, but help out with the bathing and serving out the food. It is quite confusing to sort out who is who amongst the nurses, but they should all have name badges which will tell you their rank.

There are some nurses who have undergone extra training in order to work with patients who have cancer.

Chemotherapy nurse

She is trained to look after patients undergoing chemotherapy, and will administer the drugs. She is there to talk to, and give support during what can be a difficult period, as some of the drugs have unpleasant side-effects.

Mastectomy nurse

She is trained to look after the emotional and practical problems of breast cancer patients. Apart from sorting out a suitable prosthesis, she will offer support before the operation, afterwards, and during convalescence, and will be on hand to help with any worries.

If you are having radiotherapy you will also meet the staff who work the radiotherapy equipment.

Radiographer

She has undergone training in the use of the machines that give radiotherapy treatment. You will meet her each time you come for treatment; she operates the machines.

CHAPTER 54

Alternative medicine

To be told that one has cancer is devastating; learning that it is incurable is even worse. At such times it is natural to look for solace and many turn to alternative or fringe medicine or to 'new' techniques for which unproven claims have been made. We have all heard of patients who have gone around the world looking for some 'expert' who can apparently cure cancer. Unfortunately, such quests nearly always end in failure and the cost is high in financial terms, physical distress and dashed hopes.

Unconventional or alternative medicine has become increasingly popular in both Europe and the USA. This is partly because of the failure of doctors to cure cancer and partly a rebellion against the increasing complexity of medicine. The idea of a simple, natural cure for cancer which has no unpleasant side-effects is very appealing. The promise of a chance of cure when doctors have 'given-up' is even more so.

However, such 'fringe' approaches to cancer have to be looked at with an open mind. Most such treatments rely on:

- Diet—usually vegetarian.
- Vitamin and mineral supplements—given in very high doses.
- Natural treatments—laetril or mistletoe extract for example.
- Enemas to cleanse the body—often using coffee.
- Relaxation therapy and tumour imaging.

For most patients some or all of these approaches will be recommended at once. No treatment, even natural ones, are without problems and many patients find this type of regime difficult to stick to. The diets are often *very* difficult for someone with advanced cancer to maintain: they already have little or no appetite and large amounts of vegetarian food may prove impossible. For patients with partial bowel obstruction they may be positively dangerous—the large amount of roughage increasing the risk of complete obstruction. High dose vitamins (especially vitamin C) cause diarrhoea and some drugs (such as laetril) are poisonous in high doses.

Many cancer patients going to an alternative medicine centre feel a great psychological boost—they perceive a chance of cure and feel they can do something for themselves. Unfortunately, when they return home there is often little help and support and if the cancer gets worse, as is usually the case, they feel let down and depressed. Even more depressing, because they have been told that cure is in their own hands, they feel that they have let themselves and their family down.

If you do explore alternative medicine treatments, remember that you will not be able to cure the cancer without help. You can only try your hardest, with your doctors, nurses and any other helpers—progression of cancer is **never** caused by your failure. As well as doing everything to overcome cancer, it is as well to remember that you owe it to yourself to make the most of what you have. Breaking a strict and unpleasant diet, for a special treat, will not make the difference to curing your cancer, but it might make life worth living!

If you are considering alternative medicine:

- Discuss it with your doctors.
- Approach it, and the claims made, with an open mind.
- Ask about problems associated with the treatment.
- Ask what it costs.
- Talk to people who have had similar treatment.
- Try and find out if it has been properly tested—stories of wonder cures are unreliable.
- Never, never feel that failure to cure cancer is your own fault. This is irrational; no-one would be blamed for dying of appendicitis; cancer is a 'natural' illness that has been known about for over 2000 years. It is just not within our power to simply cure it by ourselves.

Drugs commonly used to treat cancer

Drug	Method by which it is given	Common side-effects (those in capitals are commonly troublesome)

Alkylating agents. (A large group of drugs that react chemically with DNA—the genetic material in a cell controlling its division and function.)

Drug	Method by which it is given	Common side-effects (those in capitals are commonly troublesome)
BCNU	Into a vein	NAUSEA AND VOMITING, RISK OF INFECTION or BRUISING and BLEEDING, pain at site of injection, infertility.
Busulphan	By mouth	RISK OF INFECTION or BRUISING and BLEEDING, infertility, skin pigmentation.
CCNU	By mouth	NAUSEA AND VOMITING, risk of infection and bruising and bleeding, infertility.
Chlorambucil	By mouth	Risk of infection and bruising and bleeding, infertility.
Chlorozotocin	Into a vein	Risk of infection and bruising and bleeding, nausea and vomiting, infertility.
Cisplatin	Into a vein	NAUSEA AND VOMITING, risk of infection and bruising and bleeding, kidney damage if not given carefully with fluids, hearing loss for high tones, diarrhoea.

Drug	Method by which it is given	Common side-effects (those in capitals are commonly troublesome)
Cyclophosphamide	Into a vein or by mouth	Nausea and vomiting, bladder irritation (cystitis), sterility, loss of hair, sore mouth, risk of infection or bruising and bleeding.
DTIC	Into a vein	Risk of infection or bruising and bleeding, NAUSEA AND VOMITING, pain at injection site, temperature, infertility.
Mephalan	By mouth	Risk of infection or bruising and bleeding, infertility.
Methyl CCNU	By mouth	Risk of infection or bruising and bleeding, NAUSEA AND VOMITING, infertility.
Mustine	Into a vein	NAUSEA AND VOMITING, pain at site of injection, risk of infection or bruising or bleeding, infertility, HAIR LOSS.
Streptozotocin	Into a vein	Risk of infection or bruising and bleeding, nausea and vomiting, pain at injection site.
Thiotepa	Into a vein	Risk of infection or bruising and bleeding, nausea and vomiting, infertility.

Antibiotic group. (A group of drugs each of which is produced by different strains of bacteria. However, they only have a very weak effect against bacterial but can kill tumour cells.)

Actinomycin D	Into a vein	NAUSEA AND VOMITING, risk of infection or bruising and bleeding, pain at injection site, sore mouth.

Drug	Method by which it is given	Common side-effects (those in capitals are commonly troublesome)
Adriamycin	Into a vein	Nausea and vomiting, risk of infection or bruising and bleeding, pain at injection site, heart damage if an *excessive* total dose is given, COMPLETE HAIR LOSS.
Bleomycin	Into a vein, under the skin by injection, into a muscle by injection	Temperature and shivering, skin pigmentation and thickening, lung damage if an excessive total dose is given, hair loss.
Daunorubicin	Into a vein	Nausea and vomiting, risk of infection or bruising and bleeding, pain at injection site, heart damage if *excessive* total dose is given, COMPLETE HAIR LOSS.
Mithramycin	Into a vein	Risk of infection or bruising and bleeding, temperature, pain at injection site.
Mitomycin C	Into a vein	Risk of infection or bruising and bleeding, pain at injection site, nausea and vomiting, hair loss.
Mitozantrone	Into a vein	Risk of infection and bruising and bleeding, nausea and vomiting.

Antimetabolites (Drugs that intefere with DNA production).

Drug	Method	Side-effects
Cytosine arabinoside	Into a vein	Risk of infection, bruising or bleeding, sore mouth.
5-Fluorouracil	Into a vein, occasionally by mouth	Risk of infection, bruising or bleeding, nausea and vomiting, sore mouth, hair loss.
6-Mercaptopurine	By mouth	Risk of infection, bruising and bleeding.

Drug	Method by which it is given	Common side-effects (those in capitals are commonly troublesome)
Methotrexate	Into a vein or by mouth	Risk of infection, bruising or bleeding, sore mouth, kidney damage when in high doses.

Mitotic inhibitors (Drugs that intefere directly with cell division.)

Vinblastine	Into a vein	Risk of infection or bruising and bleeding, pain at site of injection, numbness and tingling of hands and feet.
Vincristine	Into a vein	NUMBNESS AND TINGLING OF HANDS AND FEET, pain at site of injection, loss of hair.
Vindesine	Into a vein	Risk of infection or bruising and bleeding, NUMBNESS AND TINGLING OF HANDS AND FEET, pain at injection site, loss of hair.

Miscellaneous. (Drugs working in various ways not included in the preceding main groups.)

Asparaginase	Into a vein	ALLERGIC REACTIONS, TEMPERATURE, sleepiness, high blood sugar.
Etoposide	Into a vein, by mouth	Risk of infection or bruising and bleeding, LOSS OF HAIR, nausea and vomiting.
Hexamethylmel-amine	By mouth	NAUSEA AND VOMITING, risk of infection or bruising and bleeding.
Hydroxyurea	By mouth	Risk of infection or bruising and bleeding, nausea and vomiting.

Other helpful books

GENERAL BOOKS

Conquering Cancer (1981)

> Israel,
> Pelican

Cancer: the Facts (1980)

> Sir Ronald Bodley Scott,
> Oxford University Presss

Coping with Cancer (1980)

> U.S. Department of Health, and Human Services,
> National Cancer Institute,
> Bethesda,
> Maryland 20205,
> USA

Cancer Care: A Personal Guide (1979)

> Harold Glucksberg and Jack Singer,
> The John Hopkins University Press,
> Baltimore,
> USA

You Can Fight Cancer and Win (1977)

> J. Brody and A. Hollets,
> Times Books Inc.,
> New York,
> N. Y. 10016,
> USA

SPECIFIC TUMOURS

You and Leukaemia: A Day at a Time (1978)
  (specifically for children)

  Lynn Baker,
  W. B. Saunders Co.

Breast Cancer: The Facts (1981)

  Michael Baum,
  Oxford University Press

The Breast Cancer Digest (1980)

  U.S. Department of Health, and Human Services,
  National Cancer Institute,
  Bethesda,
  Maryland 20205,
  USA

What Every Woman Should Know about Breast Cancer (1976)

  J. Newman,
  Major Books,
  Canoga Park,
  Ca. 91304,
  USA

Your Breast and its Care (1976)

  T. Shantha,
  Frederick Fells Inc.,
  New York,
  N.Y. 10016,
  USA

A Book for Parents of Children with Leukaemia (1975)

E. Johnson and M. Miller,
Hawthorn Books Inc.,
New York,
N. Y. 10016,
USA

Living with Lung Cancer: a Reference Book for People with Lung Cancer and their Families (1977)

B. Cox, D. Carr, and R. Lee,
Schmidt Printing Inc.,
Rochester,
MN 55901,
USA

Lung Cancer: the Facts (1984)

Chris Williams,
Oxford University Press

Living with a Colostomy (1981)

Margaret Schindler,
Thorsons Publishers Ltd.,
Wellingborough

Breast Cancer (1979)

Carolyn Foulder,
Pan Books,
London

Children with Cancer: a Handbook for Families and Helpers (1979)

M. Parker,
Callill

See various associations (page 311) for leaflets on individual tumours.

PREVENTION

Preventing Cancer: What You Can Do to Cut Your Risks by up to 50% (1978)

Elizabeth Whelan,
Sphere Books Ltd.,
London

Where can cancer patients and their families get help?

BRITAIN

BACUP British Association of Cancer United Patients

> 121/123 Charterhouse Street,
> London EC1M 6AA
>
> Telephone: administration 01-608 1785, cancer information service 01-608 1661

Bacup is a new organization that will provide information and support to patients with cancer. Based in London, it runs a telephone and postal information service, as well as publishing information booklets and leaflets.

C.A.R.E. Cancer Aftercare and Rehabilitation Society

> Sec. G.W. Poole,
> Lodge Cottage,
> Church Lane,
> Timbsbury, Bath
>
> Telephone: 0761 70731.

A self-help group of ex-cancer patients and their friends who help cancer patients to return to a normal life. Branches have been formed in Hastings, Huddersfield, London, Worthing, and Edinburgh.

Cancer link

46A Pentonville Road, London N1 9HF

Telephone: 01-833-2451

This is an organization who will provide written information on cancer and self-help groups.

Cancer Research Campaign

2 Carlton House Terrace,
London SW1Y 9AR

Telephone: 01–930 8972.

Supports cancer research and cancer units in various parts of the country. Has over 900 local branches throughout the country. Main aim is to promote research.

Colostomy Welfare Group

38–39 Eccleston Square,
London SW1V 1PB.

Telephone: 01–828 5175.

Aims to help the mental, physical, and spiritual adjustment of those who have had or are about to have a colostomy. All officers of the association have colostomies and can give advice from personal experience. Home and hospital visiting is an important aspect of their work. This group has branches in various parts of the country.

CRUSE—The national organization for the widowed and their children

Cruse House,
126 Sheen Road,
Richmond,
Surrey TW9 1UR

Telephone: 01–940 4818 (9047)

Offers a counselling service to help with the emotional difficulties of bereavement. A network of local branches exists throughout the country.

Ileostomy Association of Great Britain and Ireland

Central Office,
1st Floor,
23 Winchester Road,
Basingstoke RG21 1UE

Telephone: 0256 21288

A mutual aid association for those with a permanent ileostomy. Their main object is to help people with an ileostomy resume a full life as soon as possible. They will visit patients in their home or hospital. There are over 50 divisions throughout the country.

Imperial Cancer Research Fund

P.O. Box 123,
Lincoln's Inn Fields,
London WC2A 3PX

Telephone: 01–242 0200

This organization is concered with cancer research and in addition to running two large research centres funds projects in other hospitals and laboratories.

Leukaemia Research Fund

43 Great Ormond Street,
London WC1N 3JJ

Telephone: 01–405 0101

Exists to encourage, promote, and assist research into leukaemia
and similar blood disorders. Supports research in over 40 centres
in Britain. There are 160 local branches throughout the country.
Does publish some information leaflets for patients with lymphomas and leukaemias.

The Leukaemia Society

186 Torbay Road,
Rayners Lane,
Harrow,
Middlesex HA2 9QL

Telephone: 01–868 4107

The society was formed by parents, some of whom had leukaemic children, with the object of helping others in the same
position. Membership is now open to adult sufferers and their
families. Help is available in different parts of Britain.

Malcolm Sargent Cancer Fund for Children

Administrative Office,
6 Sydney Street,
London SW3 6PP

Telephone: 01–352 6884

Exists to give financial aid and support to children suffering
from cancer and their families, either in their own homes or in
hospital. An application for a grant is made by the GP, social
worker, or district nurse and money is available for a wide range
of needs. In addition to individual grants the fund maintains
its own social workers in Belfast, Birmingham, Edinburgh,
Liverpool, London, Manchester, and Newcastle.

Marie Curie Fund

> Head Office,
> 124 Sloane Street,
> London SW1Y 9BP
>
> Telephone: 01–730 9157

The foundation is mainly concerned with providing skilled nursing care to cancer patients. This is available through eleven residential nursing homes and a nationwide home nursing service.

The Mastectomy Association

> 25 Brighton Road,
> South Croydon,
> Surrey,
> CR2 6EA
>
> Telephone: 01–654 8643

This association is a group of women who have had a mastectomy and who are willing to talk with, and reassure other women who have recently had a breast removed. The association is nationwide but is centrally organized.

National Association of Laryngectomy Clubs

> 39 Eccleston Square,
> London SW1V 1PB
>
> Telephone: 01–834 2857

The basic aim of the laryngectomy club is to give patients the opportunity to meet and practice speaking in a sympathetic environment. It also gives support for those about to undergo an operation or those who are recovering from surgery.

National Society for Cancer Relief

Michael Sobell House,
30 Dorset Square,
London NW1 6QL

Telephone: 01–402 8125

The main object is to give practical help to cancer sufferers in need. Much of this assistance takes a financial form. Special grants are given to help pay heavy debts, fuel bills, nursing and convalescent home fees, day and night nursing, fares for treatment and relatives for visiting. Application is made via the hospital social work service, social services departments, and community nursing services. They also support a number of Macmillan continuing care units and their home care services.

Stoma Advisory Service

Abbott Laboratories Ltd.,
Queenborough,
Kent

Telephone: 07956 3371

Although run by a manufacturer this group will provide independent advice and publishes useful booklets.

Tenovus Cancer Information Centre

College Building,
University Place,
Splott,
Cardiff CF1 1SA

Telephone: 0222 483500

This centre was set up to inform the public about cancer. It is associated with Tenovus, a group supporting cancer research.

The Compassionate Friends

25 Kingsdown Parade,
Bristol B56 5UE

Telephone: 0272 47316

This is an organization of bereaved parents who through their own experience offer help to other bereaved parents.

The Urinary Conduit Association

c/o L. Kennifick,
Christie Hospital and Holt Radium Institute,
Wilmslow Road,
Withington,
Manchester 20

Provides information for patients who have had a urinary diversion.

Wessex Cancer Trust

Royal South Hants Hospital,
Graham Road,
Southampton SO9 4PE

Telephone: 0703 34288 (Ext. 447/448)

An independent charity established to raise money for cancer care and research in the Wessex region. It operates as an 'umbrella' organization for the region, promoting research, care of cancer sufferers as well as public education.

Women's National Cancer Control Campaign

1 South Audley Street,
London W1Y 5DQ

Telephone: 01–499 7532/4

This group promotes measures for the early detection of cancers of the cervix and breast by health education and screening programmes.

Glossary

TECHNICAL TERMS EXPLAINED

Ablative therapy
A treatment to totally remove or eradicate part of the body.

Adenocarcinoma
A cancer starting in glandular tissue.

Adjuvant therapy
A secondary treatment which usually follows surgery and involves chemotherapy or radiotherapy.

Adjuvant treatment
The use of treatment (usually chemotherapy) after a cancer has been completely removed. This is done when there is a high chance that the cancer will return because microscopic collections of cells have spread to other parts of the body.

Adrenalectomy
Removal of the adrenal glands.

Aetiology
The study of the cause of a disease.

Alopecia
Loss of hair which can be caused by some types of chemotherapy and radiation to the scalp. It is nearly always temporary.

Amenorrhoea
Loss of normal menstruation or periods.

Anaemia
Lack of red cells in the blood which causes tiredness, shortness of breath, and pallor.

Analgesic
Medicine given (by mouth, injection, or suppository) to control pain.

Androgen
A male hormone.

Antibody
A protein produced by the body which can attack or seek out a specific protein or structure in the body.

Aspirate
To suck off fluid with a syringe.

Astrocytoma
The commonest cancer that develops in the brain in adults.

Axilla
The armpit.

Benign
A term used to describe a tumour or tissue which is not malignant or cancerous and which, therefore, does not spread.

Bilateral
Pertaining to both sides.

Biopsy (page 21)
The surgical removal of a piece of tissue for examination under a microscope.

Blood count
A test measuring the number of red cells, white cells, and platelets there are in a blood sample.

Body scan
Another name for a CAT scan—a special X-ray that gives very detailed pictures.

Bone marrow
Spongy tissue in the middle of bones that makes blood cells.

Bone marrow biopsy and aspiration (page 53)
The removal of a small amount of bone marrow for examination under a microscope. This is done by pushing a fine needle (after local anaesthetic) into the pelvis or the breast bone.

Brain scan (page 52)
Way of examining the brain after injecting a small amount of a radioactive 'dye'.

Bronchoscopy (page 64)
Examination of the air passages with a flexible instrument called a bronchoscope.

BSE
Breast self-examination (page 13).

Cancer
A general term for more than 100 diseases where there is uncontrolled growth of cells which spread and, if untreated, eventually lead to death.

Carcinogen
A substance that can cause or help cause cancer.

Carcinoma
A cancer that develops from cells called epithelial cells. These cells are present in the skin, lungs, glands, gastrointestinal tract, and urinary tract. Cancers that develop in these sites are called carcinomas and are the commonest type of cancer.

CAT scan (page 47)
A computerized X-ray system that gives very detailed pictures.

Chemotherapy (Chapter 12)
The use of drugs to treat cancer.

Cervical smear
Scraping of cells from the neck of the womb (cervix) for examination under a microscope.

Cervix
Neck of the uterus or womb.

Cobalt therapy
Radiotherapy (Chapter 11) using radiation from a cobalt machine.

Colonoscopy (page 60)
The use of a flexible instrument to examine the entire large bowel.

Colostomy (page 291)
An operation to bring the bowel (colon) up to the abdominal wall so that stool may be collected in a special bag.

Colposcopy
Examination of the neck of the womb with a magnifying instrument passed into the vagina.

Combination chemotherapy (Chapter 12)
The use of several drugs given together to treat cancer.

Combined modality treatment
The use of more than one type of anti-cancer treatment (surgery, radiotherapy, and chemotherapy) together.

Craniopharyngioma
A tumour of the pituitary gland at the base of the brain.

CT scan *see* CAT scan

Cyst
A closed cavity or sac that contains liquid or semi-solid material.

Cystoscopy (page 154)
Use of an instrument passed through the passage from the bladder to examine the inside of the bladder.

DNA
The genetic material in the centre of a cell which controls its growth, division, and function.

Dysuria
Pain on passing urine.

Endocrine gland
Glands that secrete hormones into the bloodstream.

Endocrine therapy
The use of hormones to treat a disease.

Endometrium
Lining of the womb that is shed with each period.

Endoscopy
The use of a hollow instrument to examine the inside of different parts of the body.

Epidemiology
The study of the geographic distribution of disease.

Excisional biopsy
Total surgical removal of tissue to be examined.

Fibrocystic disease
A *benign* breast condition in which there is overgrowth of fibrous tissue often combined with formation of cysts.

Frozen section
A rapid way of examining a biopsy to see if it contains cancer; a result is available straightaway so that a suitable operation can be planned.

Gastroscopy (page 61)
The use of a flexible instrument, which is swallowed, to examine the inside of the stomach and upper part of the small bowel.

Genetic
Inherited.

Glioblastoma
A highly malignant brain cancer in adults.

Granulocytes (neutrophils)
Infection-fighting cells in the blood.

Gynaecologist
A doctor who specializes in the treatment of diseases of the female reproductive tract.

Haematologist
A doctor who specializes in diseases of the blood and bone marrow.

Haematuria
Blood in the urine.

Hepatoma
A primary cancer of the liver.

Histology
The study of tissues to diagnose disease.

Hormone
A chemical substance that circulates in the blood and causes changes in the body.

Hormone receptor assay
A special test to see if a tumour contains special receptor sites that indicate that it is likely to respond to hormonal therapy.

Hormone therapy
The use of hormones to treat a disease.

Hyperalimentation
The infusion (drip) of highly nutritious fluids containing protein and lots of calories into a vein.

Hypernephroma (page 149)
A cancer of the kidney in adults.

Hypophysectomy
Surgical removal of the pituitary gland.

Hysterectomy
An operation to remove the womb (uterus).

Ileostomy
An artificial opening between the small bowel (ileum) and the abdominal wall so that stool can be collected in a bag.

Immunotherapy
An experimental method of treatment that attempts to increase the body's own defence (immune) mechanisms against cancer.

Incidence
The rate at which a certain event occurs, such as the number of new cases of cancer occurring during a certain period.

Incisional biopsy
Surgical removal of part of a tissue to be examined.

In situ cancer
The earliest stage of a cancer where it is localized just where it started.

Intravenous (IV)
Infusion of fluid into a vein.

Irradiation
Treatment by radiation.

Laparotomy
An exploratory abdominal operation.

Laryngectomy
Surgical removal of the voice box (larynx).

Laryngoscopy
Examination of the back of the throat and voice box (larynx) using a mirror.

Larynx
Voice box situated in the upper part of the wind pipe.

Lesion
Any abnormal area (for whatever reason) in a tissue.

Linear accelerator
A type of radiotherapy machine producing a very high energy radiation.

Localized cancer
A cancer confined to the site of origin.

Local recurrence
A tumour that reappears at the site of the original tumour.

Lumbar puncture (page 252)
A test examining the fluid in the spine (CSF). After the area has been injected with local anaesthetic a needle is inserted into the spine and fluid is taken out.

Lumpectomy (tyelectomy or quadrantectomy)
Surgical removal of a cancerous lump and a portion of surrounding tissue instead of the whole organ.

Lymphatic system
Circulatory network of lymph-carrying vessels, the lymph nodes, spleen, and thymus which produce and store infection-fighting cells.

Lymph nodes (glands)
Nodules of tissue in the lymphatics that make lymphocytes and filter out unwanted substances.

Lymphangiogram (page 38)
A special X-ray test to outline the lymph glands deep in the abdomen. A contrast dye is injected into the fine lymphatic vessels in the feet and this spreads to the abdomen.

Lymphocytes
White cells in the blood that produce antibodies to fight infections.

Lymphoedema
Swelling of a part of the body because the normal lymphatics have been blocked or destroyed.

Lymphoma (page 189)
A cancer that develops in the lymph system.

Malignant
Of a tumour which is cancerous and will spread with fatal results if not removed.

Mammogram (page 13)
A special X-ray used to detect small breast cancers.

Mastectomy (page 117)
An operation to surgically remove a breast for cancer.

Medical oncology
The treatment of cancer with drugs (chemotherapy).

Mediastinum
The area of the chest containing the heart and major blood vessels.

Mega voltage radiotherapy (Chapter 11)
High energy irradiation using cobalt or linear accelerator sources.

Melanoma (page 213)
A cancer of the skin that develops from a mole.

Menarche
The beginning of menstruation at puberty.

Menopause
The cessation of menstruation.

Mesothelioma
A tumour of the lining of the lung (pleura) or of the abdomen (peritoneum) that is usually caused by asbestos.

Metastasis
The spread of a cancer from one part of the body to another. The new area of cancer is a metastasis or secondary.

Morbidity
The symptoms or effects of a disease or its treatment.

Mortality rate
The death rate.

Mucositis
Inflammation of soreness of the lining of the mouth (mucosa).

Multicentric
Having more than one centre of origin.

Mutation
A permanent change in the genetic material (DNA).

Neoplasm
A 'jargon word' sometimes used instead of cancer—means new growth.

Neutrophils (granulocytes)
Infection-fighting cells in the blood.

Node
A lymph node.

Occult tumour
A concealed or hidden tumour.

Oncology
The study of tumours (benign and malignant).

Oophorectomy (ovariectomy)
An operation to surgically remove the ovaries.

Orthovoltage radiotherapy (Chapter 11)
Low energy radiation now only used to treat superficial cancers.

Ostomy (page 290)
An artificial opening between an organ and the surface of the abdominal wall. This is done so that the excretion of the intestine (colostomy or ileostomy) or urine can be collected in a bag.

Paget's disease
A cancer of the nipple.

Palliative treatment
Treatment aimed to make a person feel better rather than to cure them.

Palpate
Feel by hand.

Pap smear (page 12) *see* Cervical smear

Paralytic ileus
Stoppage of the bowel caused by loss of normal intestinal movement.

Pathology
The branch of medicine concerned with the examination of diseased tissues.

Pectoralis muscles
The group of muscles on the front of the chest underlying the breast.

Peritoneum
The inner lining of the abdomen.

Pituitary gland
The endocrine gland at the base of the brain which controls many other endocrine glands.

Placebo
An inert substance used in controlled trials to see if a treatment is better than no treatment at all (placebo).

Platelets
Cells in the blood that help it to clot.

Pleura
The lining over the lungs.

Polyp
A benign outgrowth of tissue.

Pre-malignant
Of an abnormal area in the body that may develop into a cancer but has not, as yet, done so.

Prevalence
The total number of cases at one time in a given area.

Primary cancer
A cancer present at the site in which it developed.

Progesterone
A hormone produced by the adrenal gland.

Prognosis
A prediction of the likely course of a disease. This can only be estimated from the experiences of a lot of patients and cannot accurately predict the outcome in an individual.

Prolactin
A pituitary hormone that stimulates milk production.

Prophylactic
Of a treatment designed to prevent a disease.

Prosthesis
A specially manufactured replacement to functionally and cosmetically take the place of a part of the body that has been surgically removed. The most common are artificial breasts after mastectomy and artificial limbs.

Radiation or **radiotherapy** (see Chapter 11)
A way of damaging or killing cancer cells by using a beam of radiation.

Radiation therapist (radiotherapist)
A doctor specializing in the treatment of cancer with radiation.

Radical mastectomy (Halsted)
An extensive mastectomy that includes removal of some of the muscles on the chest wall.

Radioactive implants (page 78)
The placing (implanting) of a radioactive source in the body. This is put close by a cancer and gives it a very high dose of radiation and is then removed.

Radioresistant
A tumour that does not shrink when treated with doses of radiation that can be tolerated by surrounding tissues.

Radiosensitive
A cancer that shrinks or can be eradicated by a dose of radiation that is tolerated by nearby tissues.

Reconstructive mammaplasty
The rebuilding of a breast by plastic surgery.

Relapse (recurrence) (page 259)
The regrowth of a cancer after it has been removed or has responded to treatment.

Remission (page 259)
Shrinkage of a tumour. This may be partial or complete, but does not necessarily indicate cure.

Sarcoma
Cancers that develop in the body's supporting tissues (bone, cartilage, muscle, fat, tendons) and the tissue between organs.

Side-effects
Unwanted and sometimes unpleasant reactions to treatment that are usually temporary though some may be permanent.

Sigmoidoscopy (page 59)
A visual examination of the rectum and last part of the large bowel using a straight metal tube called a sigmoidoscope.

Simple mastectomy (total mastectomy)
Surgical removal of the breast tissue only.

Staging
The systematic investigation of the extent of spread of tumour in order to decide what treatment is best. The amount of tumour spread is described as the disease stage.

Steroids
A group of naturally occurring compounds that may act as hormones.

Stomatitis
Inflammation or soreness of the mouth.

Subcutaneous mastectomy
Surgical removal of the internal breast tissue, leaving the skin and nipple; used as a prophylactic measure.

Supraclavicular
Of the area above the clavicle (collar bone). Usually used to refer to lymph nodes at this site.

Systemic
Refers to the whole body; hence systemic treatment treats the whole body.

Tyelectomy (lumpectomy)
Surgical removal of a lump with a portion of surrounding tissue instead of the whole organ.

Therapy
A treatment for a disease.

Tomograms (page 44)
Special X-rays taken to find small abnormalities.

Toxicity
The side-effects of a treatment.

Tumour
A swelling or mass of tissue in any part of the body. It may be cancerous or benign.

Ulcer
An erosion in a surface membrane (such as in the stomach) that may be benign or malignant.

Ultrasound test (ultrasonography) (page 45)
The use of a very high frequency sound (which the ear cannot hear) to look inside the body.

Xeroradiograph
A special X-ray of the breast.

Index

335

338

340